Artificial Nutrition and Hydration and the Permanently Unconscious Patient

D1188613

Artificial Nutrition and Hydration and the Permanently Unconscious Patient

The Catholic Debate

Ronald P. Hamel
James J. Walter
Editors

GEORGETOWN UNIVERSITY PRESS/WASHINGTON, D.C.

As of January 1, 2007, 13-digit ISBN numbers have replaced the 10-digit system.
13-digit   10-digit
Paperback: 978-1-58901-178-6   Paperback: 1-58901-178-3
Georgetown University Press, Washington, D.C. www.press.georgetown.edu

Library of Congress Cataloging-in-Publication Data

    Artificial nutrition and hydration and the permanently unconscious patient : the Catholic
debate / edited by Ronald P. Hamel, James J. Walter.

    p. ; cm.

    Includes bibliographical references and index.

    ISBN-13: 978-1-58901-178-6 (pbk. : alk. paper)

    ISBN-10: 1-58901-178-3 (pbk. : alk. paper)

    1. Medical ethics.   2. Coma—Patients—Religious aspects—Catholicism.   3. Loss of
consciousness.   4. Fluid therapy—Moral and ethical aspects.   5. Religion and medicine.
6. Euthanasia—Moral and ethical aspects.   I. Hamel, Ronald P., 1946–   II. Walter, James J.
[DNLM: 1. Euthanasia, Passive—ethics. 2. Catholicism. 3. Enteral Nutrition—ethics.
4. Fluid Therapy—ethics. 5. Persistent Vegetative State—therapy. 6. Religion and Medicine.
WB 60 A791 2007]

    RB150.C6A78 2007

    179.7—dc22   2007007017

14 13 12 11 10 09 08 07   9 8 7 6 5 4 3 2
First printing

Printed in the United States of America

In memory of our parents
Arthur J. Hamel
Yvette B. Hamel
and
Joseph B. Walter
Coletta L. Walter

Contents

Introduction
The State of the Debate

The debate about forgoing or withdrawing artificial nutrition and hydration, especially regarding patients in a persistent vegetative state, dates back at least to the early 1980s. High-profile cases brought the issue to the fore and to the attention of clinicians, bioethicists, theologians, attorneys, legislators, and the general public: In the 1982 Baby Doe case, an infant with Down syndrome and esophageal atresia was denied artificial nutrition and hydration; in the 1983 Clarence Herbert case, two physicians were charged with murder for discontinuing nutrition and hydration for a patient who had suffered a profound anoxic brain injury; and in the 1983 Claire Conroy case, a nephew requested discontinuation of artificial nutrition and hydration on his elderly, demented aunt who resided in a nursing home.

Subsequent high-profile cases continued to fuel the debate while clinicians frequently struggled with decisions about withdrawing feeding tubes for the many patients who did not make the evening news or the front page of the newspaper. A good deal of literature, both secular and religious, was generated in response to the cases themselves and in response to the situations they represented. Whereas some people considered feeding tubes as another form of life-sustaining treatment subject to a burden–benefit analysis, others viewed them as a basic form of care and generally morally obligatory. Still others might permit the withdrawal of feeding tubes in patients who are imminently dying but not in patients in a persistent vegetative state (PVS). It is the latter that has become the flash point in the debate about forgoing or withdrawing artificial nutrition and hydration, as was evidenced in the recent Terri Schiavo case and in reactions to the 2004 address of John Paul II on "Care for Patients in a 'Permanent' Vegetative State." It is the papal speech that is especially the focus of this volume.

What accounts for the enormous differences in perspective between those who believe that forgoing or withdrawing artificial nutrition and hydration for patients in a persistent vegetative state is morally permissible and those who do not? The major differences seem to revolve around three issues—one clinical and two ethical.

The Nature and Prognosis of Persistent Vegetative State

One of the fundamental differences between the two positions is how one thinks about persons in a persistent vegetative state. Are they dying or are they merely seriously disabled? Some people maintain that these individuals, although not dying in the same sense as someone with terminal cancer, do have a fatal pathology that would lead to their death if they do not receive medical intervention (similar to patients with kidney failure who require dialysis). They believe artificial nutrition and hydration in such patients represents a form of life-sustaining treatment. Forgoing or withdrawing this medical intervention would be an instance of "allowing the patient to die," and, therefore, consistent with the Catholic moral tradition. Discontinuing artificial nutrition and hydration is the cessation of an intervention that will not improve the patient's condition or restore the person to health.

Others, however, do not regard the person in a persistent vegetative state as dying but as seriously disabled. They believe artificial nutrition and hydration is a form of basic care due to any human being, just like bathing, and it is not a life-sustaining treatment. Forgoing or withdrawing this type of care in a non-dying individual would be the direct cause of his or her death and would be an instance of unjustified killing. It would constitute euthanasia by omission.

Other concerns relating to the nature of persistent vegetative state that account for the differing perspectives have to do with the frequency of misdiagnoses, the possibility of "recovery" from PVS and what that recovery consists of, and whether persons in PVS can experience pain and suffering.

Human Life

Another fundamental difference between the two positions is how each regards unconscious biological life. Catholic moral theologians writing on this issue have a profound regard for the person in PVS. There is agreement that such individuals retain their full human dignity. No one claims that these persons are of less value because of their condition or that their lives are not worth sustaining.

Some people, however, believe that persons in PVS have forever lost their ability to pursue life's goods and life's goals and argue that it is not morally obligatory to sustain their biological existence. Furthermore, continued biological existence cannot be considered a benefit to the person and the individual has no awareness of his or her existence. Others, however, do regard biological existence—even if unconscious—as a good in itself and in need of being sustained. Some even argue that it is of benefit to others, allowing them to give of themselves in the care of this person and in the expression of human solidarity with some of the most vulnerable.

The Burden–Benefit Calculus

Central to the Catholic ethic of forgoing or withdrawing life-sustaining treatment is an assessment of the benefits and burdens of a particular treatment. When there is a proportion between benefits and burdens (as judged primarily by the patient), an intervention is deemed to be proportionate (or ordinary) and morally obligatory. When there is not a proportion between benefits and burdens, the intervention is judged to be disproportionate (or extraordinary) and not morally obligatory.

In the debate about forgoing or withdrawing artificial nutrition and hydration, some people maintain that this intervention is subject to a burden–benefit calculus. Whether it is morally obligatory will depend on the proportion of benefits and burdens to the patient in relationship to the patient's total condition. These individuals propose that all interventions are subject to such an analysis, regardless of how ordinary or basic they are in a medical sense, and that this, in fact, reflects the Catholic moral tradition. Nothing is determined a priori to be ordinary or extraordinary, proportionate or disproportionate.

Others, however, maintain that artificial nutrition and hydration are basic forms of care that are proportionate and generally morally obligatory. Exceptions may occur if the patient is imminently and irreversibly dying, that is, if the patient's death is very close at hand and nothing can be done to prevent it, or if the patient's body can no longer absorb the nutrients and fluids.

Quite often this issue is framed in terms of whether artificial nutrition and hydration are a form of medical treatment. The implication is that if artificial nutrition and hydration are not a form of medical treatment, then they are not subject to a burden–benefit analysis and should be considered as ordinary and morally obligatory. There is disagreement, however, whether this distinction appears in the tradition and whether it is morally relevant.

In addition, there are differences as to what counts as a benefit and how broadly one considers benefits. Should artificial nutrition and hydration be considered benefits solely because they achieve their physiological purpose (i.e., sustain life)? In other words, is life (continued physiological existence) without consciousness a benefit to the patient? Or should benefit be understood more broadly (e.g., alleviating symptoms, improving the patient's condition, restoring the patient to health)? Furthermore, in the assessment of burdens, is it legitimate to consider the burdens of the patient's condition (or the burdens of the patient's life as a result of his or her condition), as some argue, or may one only consider the burdens of the treatment itself? Here the discussion begins to move into quality-of-life considerations. At issue here is what is meant by quality of life and whether such considerations are at all permissible in making decisions about forgoing or withdrawing life-sustaining interventions. Differing views on this issue also help to account for the differing positions on forgoing or withdrawing artificial nutrition and hydration in patients in a persistent vegetative state.

These are the issues that lie at the heart of the debate about forgoing or withdrawing artificial nutrition and hydration for persons in a persistent vegetative state. They are the issues that run throughout this volume, which is intended to provide an overview of the debate within the Catholic community. To this end, we have chosen a representative sampling of the vast literature on the subject that constitutes various dimensions of the debate, namely, the clinical, the Catholic moral tradition, ecclesiastical and pastoral statements, theological reflection, the March 2004 address of John Paul II on the subject and response to it, and, finally, legal and public policy perspectives.

Part 1 offers clinical information about PVS and feeding tubes in the interests of basing ethical and theological reflection on sound data. Part 2 is foundational to the debate and provides two accounts of the Catholic moral tradition on the duty to preserve life and the limits to that duty on the one hand, and a reflection on seeming changes to the tradition on the other. The focus of part 3 is a range of ecclesiastical and pastoral statements that address the issue of forgoing or withdrawing treatment in general and that illustrate differing positions on forgoing or withdrawing artificial nutrition and hydration. In part 4 we present a sampling of a range of theological and ethical analyses of the issue. Part 5 focuses on Pope John Paul II's address on the subject as well as commentary on his address from a variety of perspectives. Finally, part 6 takes a brief look at two influential legal cases and the decisions and theological commentary on those cases. The concern here is with public policy.

Our hope with this volume is to document the debate about forgoing or withdrawing artificial nutrition and hydration for patients in a persistent vegetative state, to provide resources for students and scholars, and to invite theological dialogue on the issues that divide the Catholic community on this topic. There is much at stake here, even beyond feeding tubes. How we resolve the difficult questions raised here will have a direct impact on the Catholic ethic of forgoing or withdrawing life-sustaining treatment and how we care for dying persons.

We would like to thank Susan Lang from the Catholic Health Association for her invaluable assistance with various parts of this project.

Ronald P. Hamel
The Catholic Health Association

James J. Walter
Loyola Marymount University

PART ONE

Medical Perspectives

Good ethics, it is often said, begins with good facts. Unless there is a clear and accurate understanding of the issue at hand in its various dimensions, it is quite likely that moral judgments would be misjudgments or would be correct judgments only by chance. When what is at stake is human life and well-being, especially of vulnerable individuals, every effort should be made to obtain the best possible understanding of relevant factual information before making treatment decisions. Such information is also critical to the possibility of dialogue among those of differing perspectives. If there is not a common understanding of the factual dimensions of the issue, it is very difficult, if not impossible, to engage in conversation about its moral dimensions.

The first section of this volume is meant to provide some basic medical information about both persistent vegetative state (PVS, perhaps better called "postcoma unresponsiveness") and artificial nutrition and hydration (ANH). The information here affords a common point of departure for a moral assessment of forgoing artificial nutrition and hydration in patients in a persistent vegetative state because it reflects commonly accepted understandings of both PVS and ANH. Although what is provided here can be said to reflect the current consensus in the medical and scientific communities, not everyone may agree with this consensus. Disagreement, however, does not dispense with the need for factual and substantiated information about both PVS and ANH.

High-profile cases of the withdrawal of artificial nutrition and hydration in persons in PVS have consistently demonstrated serious misunderstanding on the part of the general public and the media of the nature of PVS and the use of feeding tubes. What is PVS and what are characteristics of this condition? Are individuals in this state aware? Do they have any purposeful activity? Can they suffer? Can they be said to be dying or to have a fatal pathology? Or should they simply be considered profoundly disabled? Do persons in PVS recover? What are clinical indications and contraindications for the placement and withdrawal of feeding tubes? What complications are associated with them? Are feeding tubes to be considered a form of medical treatment or basic care? From a clinical perspective, when might there be consideration of the removal of a feeding tube? What is seen to justify this ethically? When should such decisions be made?

The two articles in this section begin to offer some guidance with regard to these questions although they are by no means exhaustive. Serious study or discussion of each of these issues requires additional information.

I

Position of the American Academy of Neurology on Certain Aspects of the Care and Management of the Persistent Vegetative State Patient

American Academy of Neurology

I. The persistent vegetative state is a form of eyes-open permanent unconsciousness in which the patient has periods of wakefulness and physiological sleep/wake cycles, but at no time is the patient aware of him- or herself or the environment. Neurologically, being awake but unaware is the result of a functioning brain stem and total loss of cerebral cortical functioning.

A. No voluntary action or behavior of any kind is present. Primitive reflexes and vegetative functions that may be present are either controlled by the brain stem or are so elemental that they require no brain regulation at all.

Although the persistent vegetative state patient is generally able to breathe spontaneously because of the intact brain stem, the capacity to chew and swallow in a normal manner is lost because these functions are voluntary, requiring intact cerebral hemispheres.

B. The primary basis for the diagnosis of persistent vegetative state is the careful and extended clinical observation of the patient, supported by laboratory studies. Persistent vegetative state patients will show no behavioral response whatsoever over an extended period of time. The diagnosis of permanent unconsciousness can usually be made with a high degree of medical certainty in cases of hypoxic-ischemic encephalopathy after a period of one to three months.

C. Patients in a persistent vegetative state may continue to survive for a prolonged period of time ("prolonged survival") as long as the artificial provision of nutrition and fluids is continued. These patients are not "terminally ill."

D. Persistent vegetative state patients do not have the capacity to experience pain or suffering. Pain and suffering are attributes of consciousness requiring cerebral cortical functioning, and patients who are permanently and completely unconscious cannot experience these symptoms.

There are several independent bases for the neurological conclusion that persistent vegetative state patients do not experience pain or suffering.

First, direct clinical experience with these patients demonstrates that there is no behavioral indication of any awareness of pain or suffering.

Second, in all persistent vegetative state patients studied to date, postmortem examination reveals overwhelming bilateral damage to the cerebral hemispheres to a degree incompatible with consciousness or the capacity to experience pain or suffering.

Third, recent data utilizing positron emission tomography indicates that the metabolic rate for glucose in the cerebral cortex is greatly reduced in persistent vegetative state patients, to a degree incompatible with consciousness.

II. The artificial provision of nutrition and hydration is a form of medical treatment and may be discontinued in accordance with the principles and practices governing the withholding and withdrawal of other forms of medical treatment.

A. The Academy recognizes that the decision to discontinue the artificial provision of fluid and nutrition may have special symbolic and emotional significance for the parties involved and for society. Nevertheless, the decision to discontinue this type of treatment should be made in the same manner as other medical decisions, i.e., based on a careful evaluation of the patient's diagnosis and prognosis, the prospective benefits and burdens of the treatment, and the stated preferences of the patient and family.

B. The artificial provision of nutrition and hydration is analogous to other forms of life-sustaining treatment, such as the use of the respirator. When a patient is unconscious, both a respirator and an artificial feeding device serve to support or replace normal bodily functions that are compromised as a result of the patient's illness.

C. The administration of fluids and nutrition by medical means, such as a G-tube, is a medical procedure, rather than a nursing procedure, for several reasons.

1. First, the choice of this method of providing fluid and nutrients requires a careful medical judgment as to the relative advantages and disadvantages of this

treatment. Second, the use of a G-tube is possible only by the creation of a stoma in the abdominal wall, which is unquestionably a medical or surgical procedure. Third, once the G-tube is in place, it must be carefully monitored by physicians, or other health care personnel working under the direction of physicians, to ensure that complications do not arise. Fourth, a physician's judgment is necessary to monitor the patient's tolerance of any response to the nutrients that are provided by means of the G-tube.

2. The fact that the placement of nutrients into the tube is itself a relatively simple process and that the feeding does not require sophisticated mechanical equipment does not mean that the provision of fluids and nutrition in this manner is a nursing rather than a medical procedure. Indeed, many forms of medical treatment, including, for example, chemotherapy or insulin treatments, involve a simple self-administration of prescription drugs by the patient. Yet such treatments are clearly medical, and their initiation and monitoring require careful medical attention.

D. In caring for hopelessly ill and dying patients, physicians must often assess the level of medical treatment appropriate to the specific circumstances of each case.

I. The recognition of a patient's right to self-determination is central to the medical, ethical, and legal principles relevant to medical treatment decisions.

2. In conjunction with respecting a patient's right to self-determination, a physician must also attempt to promote the patient's well-being, either by relieving suffering or addressing or reversing a pathological process. Where medical treatment fails to promote a patient's well-being, there is no longer an ethical obligation to provide it.

3. Treatments that provide no benefit to the patient or the family may be discontinued. Medical treatment that offers some hope for recovery should be distinguished from treatment that merely prolongs or suspends the dying process without providing any possible cure. Medical treatment, including the medical provision of artificial nutrition and hydration, provides no benefit to patients in a persistent vegetative state, once the diagnosis has been established to a high degree of medical certainty.

III. When a patient has been reliably diagnosed as being in a persistent vegetative state, and when it is clear that the patient would not want further medical treatment, and the family agrees with the patient, all further medical treatment, including the artificial provision of nutrition and hydration, may be forgone.

A. The Academy believes that this standard is consistent with prevailing medical, ethical, and legal principles, and more specifically with the formal resolution passed on March 15, 1986, by the Council on Ethical and Judicial Affairs of the American Medical Association, entitled "Withholding or Withdrawing Life-Prolonging Medical Treatment."

B. This position is consistent with the medical community's clear support for the principle that persistent vegetative state patients need not be sustained indefinitely by means of medical treatment.

While the moral and ethical views of health care providers deserve recognition, they are in general secondary to the patient's and family's continuing right to grant or to refuse consent for life-sustaining treatment.

C. When the attending physician disagrees with the decision to withhold all further medical treatment, such as artificial nutrition and hydration, and feels that such a course of action is morally objectionable, the physician, under normal circumstances, should not be forced to act against his or her conscience or perceived understanding of prevailing medical standards.

In such situations, every attempt to reconcile differences should be made, including adequate communication among all principal parties and referral to an ethics committee where applicable.

If no consensus can be reached and there appear to he irreconcilable differences, the health care provider has an obligation to bring to the attention of the family the fact that the patient may be transferred to the care of another physician in the same facility or to a different facility where treatment may be discontinued.

D. The Academy encourages health care providers to establish internal consultative procedures, such as ethics committees or other means, to offer guidance in cases of apparent irreconcilable differences. In May 1985 the Academy formally endorsed the voluntary formation of multidisciplinary institutional ethics committees to function as educational, policy-making, and advisory bodies to address ethical dilemmas arising within health care institutions.

IV. It is good medical practice to initiate the artificial provision of fluids and nutrition when the patient's prognosis is uncertain, and to allow for the termination of treatment at a later date when the patient's condition becomes hopeless.

A. A certain amount of time is required before the diagnosis of persistent vegetative state can be made with a high degree of medical certainty. It is not until the patient's complete unconsciousness has lasted a prolonged period—usually one to three months—that the condition can be reliably considered permanent. During the initial period of assessment and evaluation, it is usually appropriate to provide aggressive medical treatment to sustain the patient.

Even after it may be clear to the medical professionals that a patient will not regain consciousness, it may still take a period of time before the family is able to accept the patient's prognosis. Once the family has had sufficient time to accept the permanence of the patient's condition, the family may then be ready to terminate whatever life-sustaining treatments are being provided.

B. The view that there is a major medical or ethical distinction between the withholding and withdrawal of medical treatment belies common sense and good medical practice, and is inconsistent with prevailing medical, ethical, and legal principles.

C. Given the importance of an adequate trial period of observation and therapy for unconscious patients a family member must retain the ability to withdraw consent for continued artificial feedings well after initial consent has been provided. Otherwise, consent will have been sought for a permanent course of treatment before the hopelessness of the patient's condition has been determined by the attending physician and is fully appreciated by the family.

Adopted by the Executive Board, American Academy of Neurology, April 21, 1988, Cincinnati, Ohio.

2

Feeding Tubes: Sorting Out the Issues

Myles N. Sheehan, SJ

The use of feeding tubes, especially in long-term care settings, is a touchy issue in Catholic health care. Decisions about feeding tube use can be difficult for a variety of reasons: complicated clinical situations, strong emotions surrounding these decisions on the part of families and caregivers, and conflicting perceptions of church teaching. Given these circumstances, not all will agree about the use of feeding tubes. But we can achieve much more clarity surrounding the issue than is currently the case.

Better decision making about the use of feeding tubes for artificial nutrition and hydration can be achieved by three interlocking actions:

- Considering the right paradigm for decision making
- Carefully evaluating the clinical details of the case in light of current knowledge
- Understanding church teachings

The Right Paradigm

What does "considering the right paradigm" mean? Far too frequently we allow conflicts and controversies about the use of artificial nutrition and hydration in the setting of persistent vegetative state (PVS) to influence our care decisions in other unrelated conditions. Decisions about artificial nutrition and hydration in PVS are extremely difficult to make; good people with good intentions may disagree. But the issues in PVS are not necessarily the same when one is addressing other medical conditions. PVS usually involves a young person in a tragic situation. It is ethically unsound to allow such a relatively rare condition to influence judgments and actions in the far more common cases of seriously ill patients, who are usually advanced in years and for whom the prognosis with or without a feeding tube is not good. The current tendency to allow PVS issues to prevail in feeding tube discussions is a bit like using conjoined twins as the paradigm for obstetrics. Both conditions are rare and tragic, and their management is morally and medically controversial. Extreme cases provide little insight into common ones.

Both the medical and ethical issues involved in the vast majority of cases in which the patient has a swallowing disorder, decreased consciousness, or some other reason for not being able to orally receive an adequate amount of food and water are often quite different than for cases of PVS. Regrettably, some of the recriminations around feeding tube removal in cases of PVS have polarized questions of feeding tube placement in cases that have very different prognoses. This confusion sometimes leads patients, family members, and health care professionals to take a moral stand without thinking carefully enough about the clinical details. Basing judgments on incomplete data is bad medicine and even worse ethics.

Clinical Issues of Feeding Tube Use

Both the decision to use a feeding tube and the care of a patient with such a feeding tube requires sophisticated medical knowledge, clinical skill, and ongoing medical attention. The use of feeding tubes requires clinicians to take four necessary actions:

- Weighing the indications and contraindications for feeding tube placement
- Choosing from several types of feeding tubes and selecting a method of placement
- Considering what actually occurs when a feeding tube is placed (because the tube is the only vehicle by which nutrients and fluids are administered, the details of the feeding are critical for success)
- Realistically understanding potential complications, both catastrophic and minor

For some, this review of the key clinical considerations in the use of feeding tubes and medically assisted nutrition and hydration may be more than they really want to know. But rudimentary knowledge of some of the medical issues at stake is essential for any sort of reasoned ethical approach. One cannot make ethical decisions in clinical situations without an appreciation of medical reality.

Indications and Contraindications

Feeding tubes are used when the patient has difficulty in swallowing, diminished consciousness, or a need to supplement inadequate oral intake when, for a variety of reasons, he or she cannot eat or drink enough material to maintain health or sustain life. Feeding tubes may be indicated when an individual has had a head injury, is in a coma, or has some other type of neurologic condition, such as a stroke or brain tumor, that prevents swallowing. Feeding tubes may also be used to bypass an obstruction in the esophagus or pharynx. In a severe illness, a feeding tube may allow adequate nutrition to be given to a person who is otherwise too debilitated to eat. In dementing illnesses, feeding tubes are sometimes used when individuals seem unable to remember how to eat or drink and therefore no longer swallow, even when food is placed in their mouths.

Feeding tubes are also used to prevent aspiration in a variety of conditions. Aspiration occurs when food, gastric contents, or oral secretions enter the lungs. Aspiration commonly results in pneumonia. For example, a person who has had a stroke but is otherwise awake and alert may have difficulty in swallowing; as a result, food or liquids go into the lungs rather than the esophagus and stomach. Feeding tubes do not prevent all aspiration into the lungs. Chronically ill, debilitated individuals with feeding tubes frequently have bouts of aspiration pneumonia even if they are not given any food or liquid by mouth. All individuals have some regurgitation of material from the stomach that heads toward the lungs via the esophagus. Saliva and other material from the pharynx can potentially end up in the lungs. In healthy individuals this occurrence is minor, and the normal processes of swallowing and other muscular reflexes in the pharynx and esophagus protect the lungs. But in individuals who are already ill, have diminished consciousness, or difficulties swallowing—precisely the people for whom feeding tubes may be a consideration—this natural defense may be weakened, leading to aspiration pneumonia despite the presence of a feeding tube.

Absolute contraindications to feeding tube placement include conditions in which the feeding formula or water cannot be absorbed by the body or the gastrointestinal tract is obstructed. An example is an individual with cancer that has spread to the intestines and grown so that the intestinal lumen is closed. Using a feeding tube in this situation would result in vomiting and severe abdominal pain. Other contraindications include individuals who are in such severe kidney, heart, or liver failure that the body cannot process, metabolize, or excrete the nutrients or fluids that would be given by a feeding tube. An example of a relative contraindication to beginning the use of nutrition and hydration through a feeding tube is a person in the very last stages of cancer. Ceasing to drink or eat in the last few days of life is part of the dying process. Inserting a feeding tube and administering formula and fluids runs a risk of fluid overload, the development of edema, and severe respiratory difficulties.

Types of Feeding Tubes

Once appropriate indications for the use of a feeding tube are noted, a choice must be made regarding the type. Feeding tubes come in a variety of types. Nasogastric feeding tubes are thin tubes inserted into the nostril, threaded into the nasopharynx, and then advanced down the esophagus into the stomach or, frequently, into the first portion of the duodenum. Gastrostomy tubes are inserted directly into the stomach, either surgically or, more commonly, by placing an endoscope through the skin. This latter type of type placement, commonly known as a PEG (percutaneous endoscopic gastrostomy) tube, involves passing an endoscope through the mouth and then into the esophagus and stomach, as is routinely done in the investigation of ulcers, abdominal pain, or esophageal reflux. Once the endoscope is in the stomach, the physician performing the procedure positions the lighted scope next to the front wall of the stomach. The light within can be seen as a red glow on the surface of the abdomen; it guides the placement of an incision through which a tube is placed into the stomach or advanced into the duodenum. Feeding tubes can also be placed more distally in the gastrointestinal tract. Jejunostomy tube placement can be performed either surgically or by a method similar to PEG tube placement; this tube is advanced into the jejunum.

Why would clinicians use one feeding tube rather than another? All feeding tubes are associated with some aspiration of saliva, esophageal contents, and regurgitated stomach contents. For short-term use—up to approximately two weeks—a nasogastric feeding tube can be a temporary therapeutic measure. These tubes, however, can press against the delicate lining of the nostrils and pharynx and lead to ulceration. They also can interfere with drainage from the sinuses and lead to blockage and infection. Although they are sometimes used for a prolonged period of time, the risks of ulceration and infection make them a less-than-ideal choice. Some patients must be restrained so that, in a moment of confusion, they do not pull on the tube and dislodge it.

Gastrostomy tubes are indicated when tube feeding will be needed for more than two weeks. Surgically placed gastrostomy tubes are inserted when a person has had previous abdominal surgeries or when placing the tube endoscopically would be dangerous. PEG tube placement is normally well tolerated in appropriate patients. Because PEG tubes require sedation, patients who are extremely ill or who have serious breathing difficulties can be at risk of complications from drops in blood pressure or respiratory arrest during placement. These complications are rare. Other complications that occur with PEG tube placement include perforation of the gastrointestinal tract, infection of the abdominal cavity (known as peritonitis), bleeding, and local infection at the site of the tube placement. Serious complications are uncommon.

Jejunostomy tubes are used when the patient has persistent problems with aspiration of stomach material into the lungs. In these situations, a tube is placed in the jejunum, the second portion of the small intestine. A jejunostomy tube may limit massive aspiration from the stomach into the lungs. Jejunostomy tubes require the use of different formulas than other feeding tubes (sometimes more expensive than gastrostomy tube formulas), and patients can have more difficulties with diarrhea. Jejunostomy tubes are associated with the same risks as gastrostomy tubes; they can also be placed in the jejunum through the skin by introducing a tube into the stomach and then threading it into the jejunum.

Whether placed nasally or in the stomach, duodenum, or jejunum, a feeding tube requires feeding formula and fluid prescribed by a physician and frequently based on the recommendations of a registered dietician. The feeding formulas are usually commercially prepared liquids that contain mixtures of carbohydrates, fats, proteins, vitamins, and minerals. Depending on the concentration of the solution, the fluid losses of the patient, and other considerations, additional water must be added to the feeding solution to avoid dehydration. Tube feedings can be ordered as bolus feedings (where a relatively large amount is given over a short period of time several times a day) or through a continuous drip in which the solution is administered at a precise rate for eighteen or more hours a day. The type of feeding solution and delivery depend on a number of factors. Patients who are tube-fed require careful monitoring—especially initially—of their fluid status, metabolic parameters, and overall nutritional condition. Bolus feedings can allow a person to be mobile when not being fed, but they do have a higher risk of aspiration. Drip feedings carry a lesser risk of massive aspiration but limit mobility and independence.

Aside from the small but real possibility of complications with feeding tube placement and the danger of aspiration, feeding tubes can be accompanied by diarrhea and other complications. Overemphasizing these risks would be irresponsible, however. In fact, such complications are most frequently annoyances and irritants rather than major disasters. Many patients tolerate feeding tubes and tube feeding. However, the use of feeding tubes is not carefree. Diarrhea, transient pneumonia, restraints that keep a confused patient from pulling a tube out, severely restricted mobility, and occasional clogging by pill fragments are day-to-day occurrences with feeding tubes. Feeding tubes are burdens, but the degree of burden varies from patient to patient.

Assessing the Efficacy of Artificial Nutrition and Hydration with Feeding Tubes

The ethical controversy surrounding decisions to withhold nutrition and hydration in persons in a PVS makes it clear that feeding tubes can keep people alive for years. This obvious fact does not support an extrapolation to other situations in which feeding tubes may be considered. Individuals in PVS tend to be relatively young and healthy except for the injury or accident that resulted in the vegetative state. As a result, they often have long life spans. Whether artificial nutrition and hydration offer the same benefit to those who receive feeding tubes most often—usually aging individuals who may be chronically ill or who have multiple conditions with a greatly diminished functional status—is not clear.

Not much literature exits on the efficacy of artificial nutrition and hydration in maintaining life or improving function. Two studies, however, suggest that the placement of feeding tubes is associated with a high mortality rate. The mortality rate is not a result of the tubes themselves—rather, feeding tubes are often placed in people who are dying. Published articles suggest that the outcome of artificial nutrition and hydration depends heavily on the underlying condition of those who undergo this procedure. A review of hospitalized Medicare beneficiaries who underwent gastrostomy tube placement in one year (1991) revealed a 15 percent mortality rate in the hospital and an overall mortality rate of nearly 24 percent at thirty days and slightly more than 80 percent in three years.[1] A study of Veterans Administration (VA) patients who received a PEG tube over a two-year period showed that almost a quarter of the patients died during the hospitalization in which the PEG tube was placed. Of the group of patients in this study, the median survival was only 7.5 months. The results of the VA study indicate that PEG tubes are placed in severely ill patients who have a very poor life expectancy, many of whom are terminally ill.[2] The conclusions of the study's authors demand careful reflection: "The substantial mortality rates may be reason to consider that some enterally fed patients who do not have swallowing disorders are not dying because of a lack of nutrition, but rather, lack the need to eat because they are dying."[3]

Ethical Grounding for Decision Making about Artificial Nutrition and Hydration

For Catholic health care, sound medical decision making requires good clinical judgment and a conscience informed by the teachings of the church. Appropriate sources for authoritative teaching about artificial nutrition and hydration include the *Ethical and Religious Directives for Catholic Health Care Services*, the 1993 statement "Nutrition and Hydration: Moral and Pastoral Considerations" from the United States Conference of Catholic Bishops Pro-Life Committee (see chapter 10 of this volume), and the remarks on this topic by Pope John Paul II made on October 2, 1998, during the *ad limina* visit of a group of bishops from the United States. All three documents show substantial agreement on the presumption in favor of medically assisted nutrition and hydration.

The *Ethical and Religious Directives* state, "There should be a presumption in favor of providing nutrition and hydration to all patients, including patients who require medically assisted nutrition and hydration, as long as this is of sufficient benefit to outweigh the burdens involved to the patient."[4] The Holy Father echoes the presumption in favor of nutrition and hydration. He differentiates between the right to refuse overzealous treatments that prolong dying "from the ordinary means of preserving life, such as feeding, hydration, and normal medical care." Pope John Paul's statement is similar in tone and content to the *Ethical and Religious Directives*: ". . . while giving careful consideration to all the factors involved, the presumption should be in favor of providing medically assisted nutrition and hydration to all patients who need them."[5]

Clinicians looking for guidance from these documents need to focus on their responsibility as physicians. Only physicians have the competence to make medical decisions. Neither the bishops nor the Holy Father have the competence to make a medical decision. The bishops and the pope do, however, have the responsibility of authoritative moral teaching. Thus, they consider the tradition of the church and the situation of the times when making recommendations about what is appropriate from an ethical perspective. Our times are filled with considerable challenges to respect for the dignity of the human person. These can be seen in attitudes in favor of euthanasia of the sick and elderly, for example, and in a callous lack of concern for the basic needs of those who cannot care for themselves.

All the statements mentioned above make it clear that food and water must be made available to people who can eat or drink. For those individuals who cannot eat or drink, a presumption in favor of medically assisted nutrition and hydration exists. As authoritative teachers who guard the faith, the bishops and the Holy Father must protect the value of life from conception to natural death; thus they make this presumption clear. But this does not translate into a requirement that a feeding tube be used in every clinical situation. As Pope John Paul II stated, careful consideration must be given to all the factors involved in the decision, meaning that the medical details of the case are crucial.

The word *presumption* means what it customarily means. It is not a rule without exceptions. A presumption in favor of medically assisted nutrition and hydration means that clinicians should use feeding tubes unless a good reason to the contrary, based on their knowledge and experience, exists. Creditable reasons that would overrule a presumption in favor of tube placement include:

- A medical contraindication to tube placement
- A prudent medical judgment that medically assisted nutrition and hydration would not likely change the outcome (the patient is dying from an underlying condition and tube placement would, at best, prolong the dying process or possibly even hasten death)
- A decision that the burdens of the treatment would outweigh the benefits

Thus the presumption in favor of medically assisted nutrition and hydration is not relevant when a person is in the last days of battling cancer or a terminal illness, such as severe congestive heart failure. The results of studies of Medicare beneficiaries and VA patients also suggest that the presumption has less force in persons who have a limited life expectancy because of medical illnesses and poor functional status.

Making Clinical Decisions

How does one synthesize clinical experience and church teaching into actual clinical decision making? A few rules of thumb may be helpful.

- Always make sure that persons who can swallow receive oral fluids and food. Removing food and fluids from those who can eat and drink on their own or with the assistance of another person is never appropriate.
- Do not offer medically assisted nutrition and hydration to those whose failure to eat or drink is part of the last stages of dying, such as with terminal cancer or advanced congestive heart failure. In these cases, the burdens of medically assisted nutrition and hydration are extremely high and benefit is minimal. These treatments could potentially cause premature death and increase suffering.
- Be cautious in using feeding tubes in persons with end-stage dementing illnesses or multiple medical illnesses and limited functional status. The benefits are uncertain and the burdens are not trivial.
- Use feeding tubes in situations of transient swallowing problems with a reasonable hope of recovery. For example, an older individual with moderate Parkinson's disease may, in the setting of a flu-like illness, have a severe exacerbation of Parkinson's and difficulty swallowing. This can lead to a vicious cycle in which the person cannot take the anti-Parkinsonian medication. In this setting, a feeding tube can allow for administration of medication, preservation of fluid and electrolyte balance, and recovery of function.
- The use of feeding tubes in PVS remains controversial. Because a period of time is necessary to make the diagnosis, presume the placement and use of a feeding tube at least as a trial measure to see if any recovery of function occurs.
- Remember that the presumption in favor of medically assisted nutrition and hydration is like the presumption in favor of resuscitation in the setting of cardiac arrest. It is strongly favored, but some situations exist in which it makes no sense and may be clinically wrong.

- A key factor in placing feeding tubes is informed consent. In the United States, a tube cannot be placed without the agreement of the patient or his or her surrogate. In Catholic health care institutions, a person can refuse therapy when he or she, making a free and informed decision, feels the burdens outweigh the benefits, unless withholding or withdrawing the procedure would be contrary to Catholic moral teaching.[6] Those cases in which the caregiving team believes a feeding tube is strongly indicated and that the patient or surrogate is not free or informed—or the action is contrary to Catholic moral teaching—necessitate institutional review and discussion, leading to the establishment of policy on the handling of such cases.

Struggles over Medically Assisted Nutrition and Hydration as a Sign of the Times

Discussions of medically assisted nutrition and hydration may have unfortunately kept those of us in Catholic health care from looking more carefully at the underlying issues. We live in a society characterized by powerful and contradictory tendencies. These include an increasing disrespect for life, open support for euthanasia and assisted suicide, and conversely, a highly aggressive technological approach to medical problems, especially in the care of the dying, that may provide a narrow answer but ignore the patient's greater needs. Those who care for the elderly and chronically ill, or for other patients for whom a decision about feeding tubes and medically assisted nutrition and hydration is not uncommon, must carefully examine the issues beneath the surface that can drive feeding tube placement.

We need to look more closely at how we approach feeding difficulties in our institutions. Feeding a person with dementia can be very time consuming. Some feeding tube decisions may be made because of a lack of staff necessary for hand-feeding. We should make staffing decisions and create care plans to ensure that these basic needs are met, although that will not be easy. Some nursing home administrators feel forced to push for feeding tubes out of a concern that state officials will treat weight loss and dehydration in nursing home residents with punitive sanctions. Some may make that attempt. Catholic health care, however, would do this nation a service by developing care protocols that emphasize a variety of interventions that make it clear that residents are not neglected and that ordinary means are used to provide nutrition and hydration to persons who, for a variety of reasons, have difficulty eating and drinking.

We also need to consider that difficulties with nutrition and hydration are often a sign that a person is approaching the end of life. These difficulties will not cause death. In the care of older persons with advanced dementia or other late-stage illnesses, the underlying approach should be one of palliative care. Determining whether use of a feeding tube makes sense is vital. Bringing family members into care planning is wise. Encouraging family members to assist with feeding and other aspects of palliative care can help assuage guilt and alleviate demands for technological response to the commonly expected decline that comes at the end of life.

Finally, some of these situations are ambiguous. If the care of patients was clear-cut, our decisions would be simpler. But it is not, and the church realizes that good people can only do their best. The teaching of the bishops and the Holy Father about a presumption in favor of medically assisted nutrition and hydration does not remove clinical ambiguity. Rather, it means that physicians and other caregivers need to grow in skill and competence and pay careful attention to individual circumstances, which are fundamental to making decisions for a particular patient. Efforts also need to be redoubled to provide care, comfort, and solace for people who are facing the end of life.

Notes

1. M. D. Grant, M. A. Rudberg, and J. A. Brody, "Gastrostomy Placement and Mortality Among Hospitalized Medicare Beneficiaries," *Journal of the American Medical Association,* 279 (1998): 1973–76.

2. L. Rabeneck, N. P. Wray, J. N. Petersen, "Long-Term Outcome of Patients Receiving Percutaneous Endoscopic Gastrostomy tubes," *Journal of General Internal Medicine,* 11 (1996): 287–93.

3. Grant, et al., "Gastrostomy Placement."

4. United States Conference of Catholic Bishops, *Ethical and Religious Directives for Catholic Health Care Services,* 2001, Directive 58, p. 31.

5. *L'Osservatore Romano,* October 7, 1998.

6. United States Conference of Catholic Bishops, *Ethical and Religious Directives for Catholic Health Care Services,* 2001, Directive 59, pp. 31–32.

PART TWO

The Catholic Tradition and Historical Perspectives

Any discussion of forgoing or withdrawing artificial nutrition and hydration for patients in a persistent vegetative state must ultimately return to the tradition. For almost five hundred years theologians beginning with the Spanish Dominican theologian Francisco de Vitoria (1486–1546) have addressed the moral obligation to preserve one's life and the limits to that obligation. These discussions have consistently focused on two primary considerations—the duty to preserve life and what is often referred to as the "relative norm."

The duty to preserve life is grounded in the Catholic view toward human life. Life is a gift of God, an outpouring of God's love. As such, it is deemed to be sacred. Because of its origin and nature, we have a moral duty to protect and sustain human life, although not an absolute duty. The relative norm recognizes that there are limits to the duty to protect and sustain human life. One is obliged to do only what offers a reasonable hope of some benefit and is not excessively burdensome. An assessment of the benefits and burdens of a particular means of sustaining life is conducted relative to the situation of the individual, ideally by the individual. In other words, the moral appropriateness of any intervention on behalf of a sick person should not be judged independently of the condition of that person. If the intervention is of benefit to the individual, as judged primarily by the individual, and is not excessively burdensome, then there is a moral obligation to employ it. This should be considered ordinary means. If, on the other hand, the intervention offers no reasonable hope of benefit to the patient or is excessively burdensome, then there is no moral obligation to employ it. This is considered to be extraordinary means.

The first two articles in this section, one by Michael Panicola and the other by Donald Henke, recount the historical development of the Catholic tradition on the duty to preserve life. They are in agreement with regard to the overall development of the tradition. They significantly disagree, however, in their interpretation of what constitutes a "benefit" and in the application of the relative norm, especially to artificial nutrition and hydration. The third article in the section, by Hamel and Panicola, points out two of the fundamental differences between those who argue that it may be morally justifiable to forgo or withdraw artificial nutrition and hydration in a patient in PVS and those who argue that it is not justifiable. The differences hinge on the application of the "relative norm" to artificial nutrition and hydration, and on the meaning of "benefit." For some, artificial nutrition and hydration are viewed as ordinary means (and, therefore, morally obligatory) independent of the condition of the patient. In the tradition, however, it seems that *any* intervention could be judged as ordinary or extraordinary only after an assessment of burdens and benefits to and for the patient. Furthermore, for some, the meaning of "benefit" seems to be limited to an intervention's ability to achieve its physiological purpose. The meaning of benefit in the tradition seems much broader.

The articles in this section raise significant questions. What is a proper reading of the tradition? Are both readings presented here correct? Or is one mistaken? Or does one represent a reinterpretation of the tradition, a further development of the tradition, especially with regard to nutrition and hydration? If so, how should that reinterpretation be assessed? Answers to these questions are ultimately critical to a sound and comprehensive moral analysis of the moral justifiability of forgoing or withdrawing artificial nutrition and hydration in patients in PVS.

3

Catholic Teaching on Prolonging Life: Setting the Record Straight

Michael R. Panicola

Recently there has been a lot of confusion among Catholics regarding the Church's teaching on prolonging life, especially when it comes to prolonging life with medically assisted nutrition and hydration. This was well illustrated in the nationally publicized case of Hugh Finn, a forty-four-year-old former newscaster in Louisville, Kentucky, who in 1995 suffered a ruptured aorta in a car accident near his home.[1] The lack of oxygen to the brain that Finn sustained as a result of the injury left him in a persistent vegetative state (PVS).

PVS is characterized by the loss of all higher brain functions with either complete or partial preservation of hypothalamic and brainstem autonomic functions.[2] Given the absence of higher brain activity, patients in a persistent vegetative state are completely unaware of themselves and their environment and are unable to interact with others. Yet because lower brain function is relatively intact, such patients exhibit periodic wakefulness manifested by sleep–wake cycles and have the capacity to achieve a wide range of reflex activities. As happened with Finn, PVS is frequently caused by an acute traumatic incident, either traumatic (such as a gunshot wound to the head) or nontraumatic (such as hypoxic ischermic [sic] encephalopathy). Recovery of consciousness is highly unlikely after twelve months for patients in a PVS caused by an acute traumatic incident and after three months for patients in a PVS caused by an acute nontraumatic incident.[3] The life expectancy of such patients is greatly reduced compared with the normal population. The average ranges from two to five years, and survival of ten years is extremely unusual. The length of survival depends in part on how aggressively the complications are treated. Death for patients in a persistent vegetative state is commonly brought on by an infection in the lungs or urinary tract, respiratory failure, or sudden death of unknown cause.[4]

From the time of the accident, Finn was unconscious and unable to communicate. He was kept alive by a feeding tube medically inserted into his gastrointestinal tract that provided the essential nutrients and fluids to maintain life. After being treated in an acute care facility and two rehabilitation hospitals with no improvement in his overall condition, he was transferred to a nursing home where he continued receiving medical treatment, including medically assisted nutrition and hydration. Controversy over his care arose when his wife, Michelle, with the support of his sister, sought to remove the feeding tube so that her husband could be allowed to die. Michelle noted that her decision was based on her husband's previously expressed wishes. Finn's parents and his brothers objected, however, and brought a suit to block the removal of the feeding tube. Several Virginia agencies, Virginia Delegate Robert Marshall, and Virginia Governor James Gilmore publicly agreed with the parents and brothers. In a televised address, Governor Gilmore stated that he had an obligation to protect the interests and rights of the state's most vulnerable citizens, including Finn. Yet despite the objections from the various groups and individuals involved in the case, "three different courts, including the Virginia Supreme Court, refused to second-guess Michelle Finn's decision that her husband would not want to be kept alive in a permanent vegetative state."[5] Finn finally died of respiratory failure on October 9, 1998, eight days after the feeding tube was removed.

One of the more bewildering aspects of Hugh Finn's case was the strong Catholic opposition to the removal of the feeding tube that had sustained Finn's life for three and a half years. A few nights before his death, hundreds of so-called Catholic pro-life activists held a prayer vigil outside of the nursing home where he was resting and protested that what was taking place was a blatant attack on life; that Finn could live for many years provided that he was not starved to death; that removing the feeding tube would be the real cause of death and not his underlying medical condition; that he should continue receiving medically assisted nutrition and hydration because it is a basic element of care; and that God alone should decide Finn's fate. The groundwork for the Catholic opposition had been laid earlier by Delegate Marshall, who stated publicly that removing the feeding tube was not only illegal but also contrary to "the teachings of the Catholic faith." He noted that "the law does not allow it. He's not on life support. He's not on a respirator. He's not brain dead. To me it is active euthanasia."[6]

The Catholic opposition in the case of Hugh Finn raises anew the question of the Church's teaching on the moral responsibility to prolong the lives of patients in a persistent vegetative state with medically assisted nutrition and hydration. Because PVS patients are usually able to breathe spontaneously and do not require ventilator support, the primary medical–moral issue is the continuation of medically assisted nutrition and hydration. (Whether to *initiate* this therapy for PVS patients is necessary only infrequently because the therapy is often started before the PVS is diagnosed.) Are the Catholic pro-life activists and Delegate Marshall correct in their assessment that withdrawing medically assisted nutrition and hydration from these patients is inconsistent with Catholic teaching? Do their views accurately reflect Catholic teaching on prolonging life that has developed over the course of five hundred years?

It is understandable that Catholics are concerned about how patients are treated as they approach the mystery of death, especially as euthanasia and physician-assisted suicide are gaining wider support. Such concern is misplaced, though, when the decision is whether to withdraw medically assisted nutrition and hydration from patients who have been accurately diagnosed in a PVS. Such decisions are morally justified according to Catholic teaching on prolonging life, and indeed seem most in keeping with the basic tenets of the teaching itself.

Foundational Works

Catholic teaching on prolonging life has formally evolved over the course of five hundred years from the foundational works of certain sixteenth and seventeenth century theologians to recent statements issued by the moral magisterium of the Catholic Church. Though the works of earlier Church figures were important to the formal development of Catholic teaching in this area, only after medicine increased its capacity to keep alive individuals who would previously have died did questions around the moral responsibility to use certain means to maintain life come into prominence.[7]

The first explicit treatment of what one is obliged to undergo to prolong life came from the great sixteenth century Spanish Dominican theologian, Francisco de Vitoria (1486–1546).[8] In his *Relectiones Theologiae*, Vitoria considers whether one violates the natural law obligation to protect and to preserve life if one fails to eat certain foods when sick. Vitoria replies:

If a sick man can take food or nourishment with some hope of life, he is held to take the food, as he would be held to give it to one who is sick. [However], if the depression of spirit is so low and there is present such consternation in the appetitive power that only with the greatest of effort and as though by means of a certain torture, can the sick man take food, right away that is reckoned a certain impossibility, and therefore he is excused, at least from mortal sin, especially where there is little hope of life or none at all.[9]

In reflecting on the types or quality of foods that one might be obliged to eat to prolong life, Vitoria argued that the best or most expensive foods need not be selected over more common items, even if these foods were prescribed by a physician and would prolong life twenty years more.[10] One would be excused from eating these more delicate foods because of the difficulty involved in procuring them.

Vitoria also addressed the issue of the use of medicinal drugs. Here, too, he pointed out that one is not obliged to use every possible means to prolong life:

One is not held, as I said, to employ all the means to conserve his life, but it is sufficient to employ the means which are of themselves intended for this purpose and congruent. Wherefore, in the case which has been posited, I believe that the individual is not held to give his whole inheritance to preserve his life, . . . From this it is also inferred that when one is sick without hope of life, granted that a certain precious drug could produce life for some hours or even days, he would not be held to buy it but it is sufficient to use common remedies, and he is considered as though dead.[11]

For Vitoria, the use of medicinal drugs really turns on the degree of certitude as to their effectiveness. Given the state of sixteenth century medicine, many drugs were considered experimental and as such sick persons were not morally obligated to use them, even if they provided a glimmer of hope in prolonging life.[12]

Another Dominican theologian from Spain played an important part in the historical development of Catholic teaching on prolonging life. Domingo Bañez (1528–1604) did little by way of substantively building on Vitoria's work on prolonging life, but he did introduce the terms "ordinary" and "extraordinary" into the discussion of morally obligatory and morally optional means of preserving life.[13] In considering one's moral obligation to undergo an amputation in order to prolong life, Bañez remarks:

He is not bound absolutely speaking. The reason is that, although a man is held to conserve his own life, he is not bound to extraordinary means but to common food and clothing, to common medicines, to a certain common and ordinary pain; not, however, to a certain extraordinary and horrible pain, nor to expenses which are extraordinary in proportion to the status of this man.[14]

Subsequent theologians were quick to pick up on the ordinary–extraordinary means distinction articulated by Bañez, and in a short time the distinction became firmly established in the Catholic moral tradition. In fact, the distinction is still operative today, even though some contemporary commentators have challenged its practical relevance.[15]

One of the theologians who accepted and expanded this distinction was the Spanish Jesuit theologian and cardinal John De Lugo (1583–1660). De Lugo is important to the discussion of the moral responsibility in prolonging life for three principal reasons. First, he maintained that one is morally obliged to use ordinary means to preserve life; not to do so would be equivalent to directly taking one's life. He mentioned one exception to the obligation to use ordinary means, however: One need not use even ordinary means if it provides no reasonable hope of benefit.[16] De Lugo described to a man facing certain death by burning at the stake:

> If a man condemned to fire, while he is surrounded by the flames, were to have at hand water with which he could extinguish the fire and prolong his life, while at the same time other wood is being carried forward and burned, he would not be held to use this means to conserve his life for such a brief time because the obligation of conserving life by ordinary means is not an obligation of using means for such a brief conservation—which is morally considered nothing at all.[17]

Thus, the obligation to use ordinary means to prolong life is, for De Lugo, dependent on some hope of benefit and some degree of duration.[18]

Second, De Lugo asserted that one is not morally obligated to use extraordinary means to prolong life. In making this argument, De Lugo drew a clear distinction between actively killing oneself, on the one hand, and allowing death to take place by refusing to submit to burdensome means, on the other.[19] The former is always morally wrong while the latter may be morally justified in certain circumstances. According to De Lugo, by not using extraordinary means, one does not intend to kill oneself, but rather to allow death to occur while employing only those means ordinarily used by common individuals.[20] Thus, De Lugo laid the groundwork for what is essentially the modern day distinction between killing and allowing to die.

Finally, De Lugo contended that ordinary means must be understood in the light of one's condition or state in life.[21] For instance, a religious novice who lives an ascetic lifestyle would not be morally required to return to the world and eat the same food as common persons, even if the food is necessary to improve the novice's health. Why? De Lugo claimed that what is ordinary for common persons in the world may be extraordinary for the religious novice, who in the cloister would not eat in the customary manner of common persons.[22] Thus De Lugo contextualized the meaning of "ordinary": What may be ordinary for one person in a given time and place may be "extraordinary" for another person in different circumstances.

Following the work of De Lugo, little advancement in the overall teaching of theologians on the moral responsibility in prolonging life was made. Saint Alphonsus Liguori (1696–1787) articulated the idea that the subjective level of repugnance one experiences toward the use of a means could make it extraordinary.[23] Yet, this type of subjectivity, based upon one's condition or state in life, was already present in the work of Liguori's predecessors. With the teaching on prolonging life relatively well established by the time of Liguori, subsequent treatments of the issue "were fairly standardized."[24]

The Twentieth Century

The ordinary and extraordinary means discussion received little special treatment until the mid-twentieth century, when two influential articles were published in *Theological Studies* by the American Jesuit theologian Gerald Kelly (1902–1964). In a 1950 article, Kelly examined the Catholic tradition on the moral responsibility in prolonging life decisions and summarized the traditional definitions of ordinary and extraordinary means.

> Speaking of the means of preserving life and of preventing or curing disease, moralists commonly distinguish between *ordinary* and *extraordinary* means. They do not always define these terms, but a careful examination of their words and examples reveals substantial agreement on the concepts. By *ordinary* they mean such things as can be obtained and used without great difficulty. By *extraordinary* they mean everything which involves excessive difficulty by reason of physical pain, repugnance, expense, and so forth. In other words, an extraordinary means

is one which prudent men would consider at least morally impossible with reference to the duty of preserving one's life.[25]

Kelly then asks whether one is *always* morally obliged to undertake ordinary means of prolonging life. He answers that such means need not be used if they do not offer the person in her or his condition a reasonable hope of benefit. Kelly notes that while not every theologian who addressed the issue of ordinary and extraordinary means articulated this exception to the rule, he "knows of no one who opposes it, and it seems to have intrinsic merit as an application of the axiom, *nemo ad inutile tenetur* [no one can be obliged to do what is useless]" (pp. 207–8). Thus Kelly, like some of his predecessors, was willing to admit that ordinary means may in certain situations be morally optional.

Kelly was inundated with responses to his original article. Theologians generally accepted Kelly's definitions of ordinary and extraordinary means of prolonging life. However, to eliminate some confusion, certain theologians requested that Kelly modify the definitions so that they included the notion of reasonable hope of benefit or usefulness. In a 1951 article, Kelly proposed the following modified definitions:

> In terms of the patient's duty to submit to various kinds of therapeutic measures, ordinary and extraordinary means would be defined as follows: *Ordinary* means are all medicines, treatments, and operations, which offer a reasonable hope of benefit and which can be obtained and used without excessive expense, pain, or other inconvenience. *Extraordinary* means are all medicines, treatments, and operations, which cannot be obtained and used without excessive expense, pain, or other inconvenience, or which, if used, would not offer a reasonable hope of benefit. With these definitions in mind, we could say without qualification that the patient is always obliged to use ordinary means. On the other hand, insofar as the precept of caring for his health is concerned, he is never obliged to use extraordinary means. (p. 550)

Kelly could now assert that ordinary means are always binding. The reason is he reorganized his definitions so that they did not refer solely to the ease or difficulty one experiences in obtaining therapeutic measures. Instead, they also incorporated the relative benefit or burden those measures bring to a particular patient in a given set of circumstances. Under his new definitions, he could say that a medical treatment once considered ordinary, such as medically assisted nutrition and hydration, is extraordinary *for this person* because it will be ineffective given the person's poor medical condition and dismal prognosis.

The foundational teachings on prolonging life and Kelly's specification of the meaning of ordinary and extraordinary means was given clear papal confirmation by Pope Pius XII (1876–1958) in an address delivered to an International Congress of Anesthesiologists on November 24, 1957.[26] In discussing one's moral obligation to use mechanical ventilation to preserve life, Pius XII outlined some of the major features of the ordinary-extraordinary means distinction as it had developed since Vitoria.

> Natural reason and Christian morals say that man (and whosoever is entrusted with the task of taking care of his fellowman) has the right and duty in case of serious illness to take the necessary treatment for the preservation of life and health. . . . But normally one is held to use only ordinary means—according to circumstances of persons, places, times and culture—that is to say, means that do not involve any grave burden for oneself or another. A more strict obligation would be too burdensome for most men and would render the attainment of the higher, more important good too difficult. Life, health, all temporal activities are in fact subordinated to spiritual ends. On the other hand, one is not forbidden to take more than the strictly necessary steps to preserve life and health, as long as he does not fail in some more serious duty. (p. 192)

Not only did Pius XII validate the ordinary–extraordinary means distinction in this statement, but he also illuminated an aspect of Catholic teaching on prolonging life that is important but often neglected. With a veiled reference to Saint Thomas, Pius XII suggested that human life is not the ultimate or final end of the person, but rather one's end resides in God. It is for this reason that Pius XII emphasizes that spiritual goods are higher and more important than temporal goods, even human life. Though human life is a basic and precious good, it is a limited good insofar as it is a condition for pursuing the spiritual goods of life (love of God and love of neighbor). (p. 192)

By situating the discussion of the means necessary to prolong life against the backdrop of one's ultimate end in God, Pius XII specified even more precisely the meaning of ordinary and extraordinary means. He implies that medical treatment must be evaluated in the light of the patient's overall medical condition and the patient's ability to pursue spiritual goods. Thus ordinary means are those that are morally obligatory because they offer a reasonable hope of benefit in helping one to pursue the spiritual goods of life without imposing an excessive burden; and extraordinary means are those means that are morally optional because they do not offer a reasonable hope of benefit in terms of helping one to pursue the spiritual goods of life, *or* because they impose an excessive burden on one and profoundly frustrate one's pursuit of the spiritual goods of life.[27]

The Congregation for the Doctrine of the Faith provided further confirmation of the centuries-long teaching on the moral responsibility in prolonging life in its 1980 *Declaration on Euthanasia*.[28] Addressing the issue of whether all possible means must be used to preserve life, the CDF noted that the terms "ordinary" and "extraordinary" are less clear today, and that perhaps the terms *proportionate* and *disproportionate* are more accurate. How does one assess the proportionality of means? The CDF answered that one should "study the type of treatment to be used, its degree of complexity or risk, its cost and the possibilities of using it, and [compare] these elements with the result that can be expected," taking into account one's overall medical condition and physical and moral resources (p. 263).

The CDF also remarked that one need make do only with the normal means that medicine can offer, without having recourse to established medical treatments that carry a risk or disproportionate burden. The CDF made clear that one's refusal of disproportionate treatment "is not the equivalent of suicide," rather "it should be considered as an acceptance of the human condition," a desire to avoid excessive burdens, or a wish not "to impose excessive expense" on one's family or the community (p. 263). The CDF also specified that when death is imminent, one may withhold or withdraw certain forms of medical treatment that "would only secure a precarious and burdensome prolongation of life" (p. 263).

The *Declaration on Euthanasia* establishes that Catholic teaching on prolonging life has continued largely unchanged from the time of Vitoria to today.[29] Introducing the terms "proportionate" and "disproportionate" did not significantly change the teaching. The moral norms operative in the *Declaration on Euthanasia* are some of the very same ones present in the foundational teachings of sixteenth and seventeenth century theologians.

By way of summary, the moral norms that ground Catholic teaching on prolonging life will be listed. Six moral norms emerge from the centuries-long history of Catholic teachings on prolonging life.

1. Human life is a basic and precious good which one has an obligation to protect and to preserve. However, human life is a limited good subordinated to higher, more important spiritual goods (love of God and love of neighbor).

2. One's moral obligation to prolong life through medical means is evaluated in light of one's overall medical condition and one's ability to pursue the spiritual goods of life.

3. One should be able to make medical-moral decisions for oneself. In the unfortunate circumstance that one loses decisional capacity, a designated proxy should determine what is in the overall best interests of the patient.

4. One *is* morally obliged to prolong life with medical means when it offers a reasonable hope of benefit in helping one to pursue the spiritual goods of life without imposing an excessive burden.

5. One *is not* morally obliged to prolong life with medical means (a) when death is imminent and medical treatment will only prolong the dying process; (b) when medical treatment offers no reasonable hope of benefit in terms of helping one pursue the spiritual goods of life; *or* (c) when medical treatment imposes an excessive burden on one and profoundly frustrates one's pursuit of the spiritual goods of life. One's decision not to use these types of means is not morally equivalent to killing oneself; it is a courageous choice by one to recognize higher, more important goods than the good of human life.

6. Benefit and burden are understood broadly in Catholic teaching on prolonging life to refer not just to the physiological dimension of life, but to the psychological, social, and spiritual dimensions as well.

Contrary Positions

In a way, Catholic teaching on prolonging life is fairly straightforward. Those means considered ordinary or proportionate are morally obligatory and those means considered extraordinary or disproportionate are morally optional. However, determining precisely which means are morally obligatory and which means are morally optional in concrete cases is difficult. This is especially true in cases involving PVS patients and others who cannot make decisions for themselves. A consensus is lacking among both the Catholic laity and the leaders of the church as to how far the moral obligation extends to sustain the lives of PVS patients with medically assisted nutrition and hydration.

New Jersey Catholic Conference. In its *amicus curiae* brief concerning the case of Nancy Jobes, a thirty-one-year-old woman in a PVS, the New Jersey Catholic Conference argues against the removal of medically assisted nutrition and hydration.[30] The conference states that the Catholic tradition recognizes a positive moral duty to prolong human life, and therefore nutrition and hydration, "which are basic to human life," should always be provided to PVS patients (p. 582). The conference claims that nutrition and hydration are from [*sic*] such patients "clearly distinguished from medical treatment" (p. 583). Whereas medical treatment is therapeutic and is aimed at curing disease, nutrition and hydration are directed at sustaining life and promoting the inherent dignity of the patient.

The conference maintains that nutrition and hydration do not impose an excessive burden on patients in a PVS because they cannot feel pain and that such patients actually benefit from this basic care through the preservation of their lives. Because human life is a great good and no one can directly take the life of an innocent person, the conference asserts that the removal of medically assisted nutrition and hydration from PVS patients is always morally wrong. Withholding nutrition and hydration from such patients "ultimately results in starvation, dehydration and death. It is direct. It is unnatural, as unnatural as denying one the air needed to breathe, or murder by asphyxiation" (p. 582).

If these reasons were not enough to demonstrate that withdrawing medically assisted nutrition and hydration from patients in a persistent vegetative state is an unjustifiable attack on life, the conference illuminates some of the profound social implications that would result if this type of activity was given legal sanction. First, the conference notes that allowing physicians the leeway to withdraw basic care such as nutrition and hydration from PVS patients would destroy the very ethical foundations of medicine. Second, the conference remarks that withdrawing basic care from patients who are not dying but are in a PVS is a clear statement that the patient's life has no moral value or worth. Finally, the conference holds that the practice of removing nutrition and hydration from patients in a persistent vegetative state would lead to a slippery slope. "Today food and nutrition is withdrawn from someone in a persistent comatose state; tomorrow such care is withdrawn from someone suffering from Alzheimer's disease" (p. 584).

Texas Catholic Bishops. A rather different position was marked out by the Texas Catholic Bishops in a joint statement responding to the confusion surrounding the Church's teaching on prolonging life with medically assisted nutrition and hydration.[31] The bishops start by delineating the basic moral values and the principles that are to be promoted and protected in all patient care. Among these foundational claims are principles holding that life is always a good and that every reasonable effort should be made to maintain it, but that sometimes one is beset with a medical condition that diminishes or removes one's obligation to sustain life. If the reasonable benefits to a patient from any medical means outweigh the burdens to the patient, then those medical means are morally obligatory. But if the burdens from the medical means used to prolong the patient's life are disproportionate in relation to the benefits, then those medical means are morally optional and need not be employed.

The bishops reflect specifically on PVS. They state at the outset that patients in a PVS remain human persons despite their condition. Nevertheless, they note that the PVS is a lethal pathology and that without medically assisted nutrition and hydration, PVS patients would die. What conditions make it morally obligatory to continue medically assisted nutrition and hydration for these patients? They argue that each case must be decided on its own merits, and the final decision should be based on the application of the moral values and basic moral principles outlined above "regarding the burden/benefit analysis relative to the use of life-sustaining procedures" (p. 54). For patients who cannot make decisions for themselves, they hold, treatment decisions should be made by an appropriate surrogate, and should be rendered in light of what the patients themselves would have decided.

The Texas bishops conclude by claiming that patients, including those in a PVS, must never be abandoned and should always be provided supportive nursing care in order to maintain personal dignity and hygiene. The bishops point out that *appropriate* withdrawal of medically assisted nutrition and hydration from PVS patients is not abandonment. Rather, "it is accepting the fact that the person has come to the end of his or her pilgrimage and should not be impeded from taking the final step" (p. 54). The bishops caution, however, that the withdrawal of medically assisted nutrition and hydration from patients in this condition should occur only after serious contemplation based upon "the best medical and personal information available" (p. 54).

Committee for Pro-Life Activities of the National Conference of Catholic Bishops.[32] This committee was asked by the NCCB to respond to the growing controversy around prolonging life with medically assisted nutrition and hydration. Like the Texas bishops, the committee sets forth basic moral principles. It stipulates, among other points, that human life is a fundamental human good, and that all crimes against life are always morally impermissible. It also holds that while all persons have a duty to protect and to preserve human life, the duty has limits, and persons are not obliged to prolong life by extraordinary or disproportionate means—that is, by means that offer no reasonable hope of benefit or involve excessive burdens. When death is imminent and medical treatment would only prolong the dying process, one need not submit to every possible medical means. And because death is a natural consequence of life and opens the door to eternal life, patients should accept the reality of death and prepare for death psychologically, socially, and spiritually.

Appling the basic moral principles to PVS patients in the Catholic community is difficult, the committee notes, as "some moral questions in this area have not been explicitly resolved by the church's teaching authority" (p. 709). But the committee holds that the withdrawing of all life support, including medically assisted nutrition and hydration, "not be viewed as appropriate or automatically indicated for the entire class of PVS patients simply because of a judgment that they are beyond the reach of medical treatment that would restore consciousness" (p. 710). The committee concludes that treatment decisions for patients in a persistent vegetative state "should be guided by a *presumption in favor* of medically assisted nutrition and hydration" (p. 710, emphasis added). Any decisions to withdraw medically assisted nutrition and hydration from such patients should be made by carefully examining the burdens and benefits of the treatment for the individual patients, their families, and the overall community. Medical treatment must never be removed with the direct intention of causing death, but may be removed if the treatment offers no reasonable hope of sustaining life or involves disproportionate risks or burdens. The committee adds, in closing, that its statement is not the "last word" but the "first word" on the subject, and that public discussion needs to continue so that it can be determined how best to address the complex issues surrounding PVS patients (p. 710).

Toward Consensus

Thus recent Catholic statements reach different conclusions about the obligation to provide medically assisted nutrition and hydration. The New Jersey Catholic Conference treats medically assisted nutrition and hydration as a basic element of care that should be provided to all patients regardless of their condition. The Texas bishops view it as a medical treatment subject to the same moral norms that guide decisions for other medical treatments. And the Committee for Pro-Life Activities holds that there should be a "presumption in favor" of its use. The differences among these Catholic statements indicate that the issue of prolonging the lives of PVS patients with medically assisted nutrition and hydration is a matter open for discussion within the Catholic community.[33]

Yet despite the fact that the moral magisterium has not resolved this issue and that serious disagreement exists among Catholics, two particular tenets in Catholic teaching on prolonging life suggest that withdrawing medically assisted nutrition and hydration from patients who have been accurately diagnosed in a persistent vegetative state is morally justified.

Human life is a basic but limited good. Catholic teaching on prolonging life affirms that human life is a basic and precious good that flows forth from God. The love that God has for humanity is shown most enduringly in the life of the human person who has been made in God's image. Human persons would not even exist were they not created out of and continually sustained by God's love.[34] "Life as a sign of God's love and care is sacred, has meaning because of God's love and not because of personal merit, and should be treated with dignity and respect at every stage."[35] The good of human life is not tied to functional ability or social utility, but to the very fact that it emanates from God.

It is because human life is an utterly free and unmerited gift from God that one has a duty to protect and to preserve life. Fulfilling this duty in the course of one's existence may sometimes involve seeking medical assistance and receiving medical care. However, Catholic teaching on prolonging life has always held that the duty to maintain life through medical means is limited. It ceases when medical treatment cannot offer one any hope at all of pursuing the spiritual goods of life, or can only offer one a physical condition where the pursuit of the spiritual goods of life will be profoundly frustrated in the mere effort for survival.[36] This is exactly what Pius XII means when he states:

> But normally one is held to use only ordinary means—according to circumstances of persons, places, times and culture—that is to say, means that do not involve any grave burden for oneself or another. A more strict obligation would be too burdensome for most men and would render the attainment of the higher, more important good too difficult. Life, health, all temporal activities are in fact subordinated to spiritual ends.[37]

The pursuit of the spiritual goods of life is intimately connected with human life in that physical existence affords one the opportunity to enter into communion with God through engaging others in human relationships.[38] One is able to love God in the context of human life by loving others as oneself. Yet, human life is not itself an absolute good. The good of life is a limited good precisely because it is the basis for pursuing the higher, more important spiritual goods of life.[39]

Applying this understanding of human life to PVS patients suggests that the duty to protect and to preserve their lives has ceased. Because these patients have reached a point where their ability to pursue the spiritual goods of life has been *totally eclipsed*, the best treatment is no treatment. They are beyond the reach of medical treatment (including medically assisted nutrition and hydration) and should only be provided supportive nursing care so that they may be allowed to die in relative peace without having their physical lives prolonged by unreasonable medical means. The decision to allow PVS patients to die does not imply that their lives are less valuable than others. In truth, "every human being, regardless of age or condition, is of incalculable worth."[40] Rather, the decision is based on the fact that physiological existence no longer offers these patients any hope at all of pursuing those goods for which human life is the fundamental condition (p. 350).

This understanding of human life as a limited good subordinated to the spiritual goods of life has not been embraced by everyone. Some authors argue that certain goods cannot be weighed against each other, that they are incommensurable because they are necessary for integral human fulfillment.[41] Aesthetic experience, human life, knowledge, play, practical reasonableness, religion, and sociability are all examples of incommensurable goods.[42] These goods should be recognized and respected in the context of human life. However, it is not always possible to promote all of these goods in a particular situation and thus a reasonable selection of one or another good to be more fully realized is morally acceptable. Yet, no reasonable grounds suffice for sacrificing or attacking one good for another. Incommensurable goods must all be accepted as moral realities and appreciated in every situation.

This concept of goods is problematic for two reasons. First, it fails to recognize that in fact goods often must be weighed, one against the other. Because of the limits of temporal existence, a choice for one good automatically rules out a choice for other goods. For instance, if one chooses to play a round of golf one day, one closes the door on other options, at least while one is golfing. During the round of golf, one is unable to pursue the other goods, whether it be furthering one's knowledge of the arts or strengthening one's faith commitment through attending a liturgy. This is a weighing of goods and suggests that goods are not incommensurable in reality.

Second, this concept of goods tends toward vitalism. If the good of human life cannot be weighed against other goods, then life has to be prolonged insofar as this is a physical possibility.[43] But is this right? Are there no limits to life?

Do we exist simply so that our vital physiological functions can be maintained? Or do we exist so that we can experience life, engage loved ones, interact with others, participate in society, pursue personal interests, at least at a minimal level? Accepting that human life is an incommensurable good that cannot be compared to other goods in reaching medical–moral decisions would be devastating. It would negate the rights of patients to make autonomous decisions around limiting medical care; it would lead to overtreatment whereby some lives would be prolonged way beyond what is reasonable; and it would impose a major burden on families and society to meet the demands and absorb the costs associated with caring for patients whose lives are prolonged unnecessarily. Human life is indeed always a good, as some of the supporters of the incommensurable goods theory point out, but it is a good that need not and should not be absolutized.

Treatment must offer a reasonable hope of benefit. Catholic teaching on prolonging life asserts that for a medical means to be considered morally obligatory it must offer one a reasonable hope of benefit. In assessing the potential benefit of medical treatment, several criteria must be considered. Recall the statement in the *Declaration on Euthanasia*, one should "study the type of treatment to be used, its degree of complexity or risk, its cost and the possibilities of using it, and [compare] these elements with the result that can be expected," taking into account one's overall medical condition and physical and moral resources.[44] All of these criteria coalesce in determining whether a particular medical means offers one a reasonable hope of benefit.

While it is clear that a benefit must accrue to one for a medical treatment to be considered morally obligatory, it is less clear as to what constitutes a benefit. In the medical context, a treatment is considered beneficial if it restores one's health, relieves one's pain, improves one's physical mobility, returns one to consciousness, enables one to communicate with others, and so on.[45] Catholic teaching on prolonging life recognizes all of these improvements in one's condition as benefits, but it specifies that a treatment is truly beneficial insofar as it improves one's condition to the point that one is able to pursue the spiritual goods of life at least at a minimal level without experiencing significant burdens.[46] Bishop William Bullock (Des Moines, Iowa) describes this well:

> God has given life to carry out human activities that make us better persons, serve the community and lead to eternal life with Him. Therefore, the benefit of care or treatment to prolong [the] life of a dying person, or of a person for

whom these human activities have become very difficult or even no longer possible, diminishes in proportion to what remains possible for them.[47]

This more holistic understanding of benefit is profoundly connected to the Catholic view of the human person as a physical, psychological, social, and spiritual being whose ultimate goal in life is to enter into communion with God through loving others as oneself.[48]

Applying this understanding of benefit to PVS patients suggests that medical treatment is not morally obligatory because it does not provide any reasonable hope of benefit to these patients. Though a medical treatment such as medically assisted nutrition and hydration provides the sustenance necessary to prolong the lives of PVS patients, it is not considered a beneficial medical treatment in the Catholic moral tradition because it does not restore these patients to a relative state of health. No matter how long medically assisted nutrition and hydration prolongs their lives, it will never improve their condition to the point that they can experience life in a way that enables them to pursue any spiritual goods even at a minimal level. The tragic reality is that these patients are no longer capable of receiving any meaningful benefit from medicine's efforts to keep them alive.

The holistic understanding of benefit has not been embraced by everyone. Some authors contend that the mere fact that human life can be prolonged is a benefit sufficient to justify continued medical treatment. William May, in an article coauthored with several others, argues that feeding and hydrating PVS patients "by means of tubes is *not* useless in the strict sense because it does bring to these patients a great benefit, namely, the preservation of their lives and the prevention of their death through malnutrition and dehydration."[49] Why is the mere prolongation of life itself a "great benefit"? How do patients who cannot experience life, engage loved ones, interact with others, participate in society, pursue personal interests, at least at a minimal level, benefit from having their lives prolonged? These are questions that May is unable to answer because he fails to recognize that "what is truly beneficial to us as human persons is a broad human judgment" that encompasses more than just the physiological dimension of life.[50] Catholic teaching on prolonging life has never accepted such a narrow concept of benefit as the one proposed by May. To do so would be an idolization of human life and would be an abandonment of the fundamental Christian conviction that human life is not the final end of the person. Richard McCormick sketches a "fanciful scenario" that speaks to this point: Imagine a

300-bed Catholic hospital with all beds supporting PVS patients maintained for months, even years by gastrostomy tubes. . . . An observer of the scenario would eventually be led to ask: "Is it true that those who operate this facility actually believe in eternal life?" (p. 232).

To circumvent this criticism, some authors maintain that medically assisted nutrition and hydration is not a medical treatment, subject to questions of benefit, but is a basic element of care and as such should always be provided to a patient. Robert Barry argues that medically assisted nutrition and hydration is not on the same moral plane as medical treatments because medical treatment aims at curing a clinically diagnosable condition, whereas medically assisted nutrition and hydration are responses to "the basic needs of organisms to function and grow . . . not remedies of diseases in and of themselves" (p. 232). But this misrepresents the nature of the therapy. No significant moral difference exists between medically assisted nutrition and hydration and, say, mechanical ventilation, which most everyone agrees is a medical treatment. Both are administered and supervised by medical professionals, and both are geared toward restoring a vital physiological function. As Albert Moraczewski remarks:

> Oxygen, water, and food are all necessary elements for maintaining life. If because of some current pathology, the person requires that these be supplied by technological means, then it would seem that the same moral principles can be applied to determine the respective moral obligations to initiate or continue life conserving procedures. By technological means we are circumventing an obstacle that prevents food and water (or oxygen) from entering the body in the normal manner. Hence when we cease by-passing the obstacle, the person dies from a combination of his pathology and the lack of nutrition and hydration (or oxygen).[51]

Yet even if it were determined that medically assisted nutrition and hydration are basic forms of care, the decision to initiate or continue them would still hinge on the moral norms articulated in Catholic teaching on prolonging life.[52] Even the sixteenth and seventeenth century theologians held that the taking of food could be considered extraordinary or morally optional given one's condition and present circumstances.[53] And these theologians were talking about ordinary "food," taken in everyday ways.

To be sure, decisions to withdraw medically assisted nutrition and hydration from PVS patients will be emotionally difficult for family members and medical professionals. Indeed, one may *feel*, incorrectly, as though one is killing the patient. [54] Yet so long as one's decision to remove the feeding tube corresponds with the moral norms of Catholic teaching and is not directly intended to kill the patient, one is on sound moral grounding. Such a decision, far from being morally equivalent to murder, reflects an acceptance of the limits of life and of the human condition in the end of life. And while Catholics are quick to witness to the value of life, we should be equally as quick to witness to the limits of life. This recognition of life's limits would be as clear a statement as any that we believe and trust in God who has been most fully revealed in the *life, death, and resurrection* of Christ Jesus.

Notes

1. See A. Goldstein, "'Pro-Life' Activists Take on Death: Movement Mobilizes Against Issues Such as Assisted Suicide," *Washington Post*, November 10, 1998; B. A. Masters, "Conscious of Life in the Balance: Brain-Injured Man's Divided Family Caught in Legal, Medical Netherworld," *Washington Post*, September 27, 1998; B. A. Masters, "Family Reunites as Hundreds Mourn Finn: Pastor Calls for Forgiveness," *Washington Post*, October 13, 1998.

2. Multi-Society Task Force on PVS, "Medical Aspects of the Persistent Vegetative State," *NEJM* 330 (1994): 1499–1508 and 1572–79, at 1500.

3. C. Weijer, "Cardiopulmonary Resuscitation for Patients in a Persistent Vegetative State: Futile or Acceptable," *Canadian Medical Association Journal* 158 (24 February 1998): 491–93, at 491.

4. R. S. Howard and D. H. Miller, "The Persistent Vegetative State," *British Medical Journal* 310 (11 February 1995): 341–42, at 341.

5. Masters. "Family Reunites as Hundreds Mourn Finn," p. 4.

6. R. B. Marshall, quoted in J. J. Paris, "Hugh Finn's 'Right to Die,'" *America* 179 (31 October 1998): 13-15, at 13–14.

7. D. A. Cronin, *Conserving Human Life*, ed. Russell E. Smith (Braintree, Mass.: Pope John Center, 1989), 34. This work is a republication of Cronin's doctrinal dissertation *The Moral Law in Regard to the Ordinary and Extraordinary Means of Conserving Life* (Rome: Gregorianum, 1958).

8. Some authors begin their historical sketches of Catholic teaching on prolonging life with Saint Thomas Aquinas (1225–1274), who set the parameters for the discussion. Most recognize Vitoria as the first theologian to explicitly address questions around the means to prolong life. See R. A. McCormick and J. J. Paris, "The Catholic Tradition on the Use of Nutrition and Fluids," *America* (2 May 1987): 356–61; K. D. O'Rourke, *Development of Church Teaching on Prolonging Life* (St. Louis: Catholic Health Association, 1988); and R. C. Sparks, *To Treat or Not To Treat? Bioethics and the Handicapped Newborn* (New York: Paulist Press, 1988), 85–100.

9. F. De Vitoria, *Relectiones Theologiae* (Lugdini, 1587), Relectio IX, de Temperentia, n. 1 (translated as in Cronin, *Conserving Human Life*, p. 35).

10. F. De Vitoria, *Relectiones Theologiae*, Relectio IX, de Temperentia, n. 12 (translated as in Cronin, *Conserving Human Life*, p. 36); and F. De Vitoria, *Comentarios a la Secunda Secundae de Santo Tomas*

(Salamanca, ed. de Heredia, 1952), II:II, q. 147, a. I (translated as in Cronin, *Conserving Human Life*, p. 37).

11. F. De Vitoria, *Relectiones Theologiae*, Relectio X, de Homicido, n. 35 (translated as in Cronin, *Conserving Human Life*, p. 37).

12. Sparks, *To Treat or Not To Treat?* p. 95.

13. Several authors attribute this introduction of the terms "ordinary" and "extraordinary" to Bañez. See, for instance, J. J. McCartney, "The Development of the Doctrine of Ordinary and Extraordinary Means of Preserving Life in Catholic Moral Theology Before the Karen Quinlan Case," *Linacre Quarterly* 47 (August 1980): pp. 215–24; McCormick and Paris, "The Catholic Tradition on the Use of Nutrition and Fluids," p. 358; J. J. Mulligan, "The Catholic Tradition on Means of Sustaining Life," in *Scarce Medical Resources and Justice* (Braintree, Mass.: Pope John Center, 1987), 74–87, at 78; and ref. 8, O'Rourke, *Development of Church Teaching on Prolonging Life*, 21, n. 6.

14. D. Bañez, *Scholastica Commentaria in Partem Angelici Doctoris S. Thomae* (Duaci, 1614–1615), Tom. IV, Decisiones de Jure et Justitia, in II II, q. 65, a. I (translated as in Cronin, *Conserving Human Life*, p. 42).

15. See T. L. Beauchamp and J. F. Childress, *Principles of Biomedical Ethics*, 4th ed. (New York: Oxford University Press, 1994), 196–202; and President's Commission for the Study of Ethical Problems in Medicine and Biomedical and Behavioral Research, *Deciding to Forego Life-Sustaining Treatment* (Washington, D.C.: U.S. Government Printing Office, March 1983), 82–90.

16. Cronin, *Conserving Human Life*, pp. 53–55.

17. John De Lugo, *Disputationes Scholasticae et Morales* (ed. nova, Parisiis, Vivès, 1868–1869), vol. VI, *De Iustitia et Iure*, Disp. X, sec. I, n.30 (translated as in Cronin, *Conserving Human Life*, 54).

18. See ref. 7, Cronin, *Conserving Human Life*, p. 54.

19. G. M. Atkinson, "Theological History of Catholic Teaching on Prolonging Life," in *Moral Responsibility in Prolonging Life Decisions*, ed. D. G. McCarthy and A. S. Moraczewski (St. Louis: Pope John Center, 1981), 95–115, at 101; and ref. 7, Cronin, *Conserving Human Life*, p. 55.

20. De Lugo, *Disputationes Scholasticae et Morales*, vol. VI, *De Iustitia et lure*, Disp. X, sec. I, n.36 (translated as in Cronin, *Conserving Human Life*, p. 55).

21. Cronin, *Conserving Human Life*, p. 55.

22. De Lugo, *Disputationes Scholasticae et Morales*, vol. VI, *De Iustitia et lure*, Disp. X, sec. I, n.36 (translated as in Cronin, *Conserving Human Life*, p. 55).

23. Atkinson, "Theological History of Catholic Teaching on Prolonging Life," in *Moral Responsibility in Prolonging Life Decisions*, p. 103.

24. Cronin, *Conserving Human Life*, p. 66.

25. G. Kelly, "The Duty of Using Artificial Means of Preserving Life," *Theological Studies* 11 (June 1950): 203–20; G. Kelly, "The Duty to Preserve Life," *Theological Studies* 12 (December 1951): 550–56.

26. Pius XII, "The Prolongation of Life," in *Critical Choices and Critical Care*, ed. K. W. Wildes (Netherlands: Kluwer Academic Press, 1995), 189–96.

27. O'Rourke, *Development of Church Teaching on Prolonging Life*, p. 5; J. J. Walter makes a similar assessment of morally obligatory and morally optional means of prolonging life, though under a quality of life approach and not an ordinary–extraordinary means approach, in "The Meaning

and Validity of Quality of Life Judgments in Contemporary Roman Catholic Medical Ethics," in *Quality of Life: The New Medical Dilemma*, ed. J. J. Walter and T. A. Shannon (New York: Paulist Press, 1990) 78–88. See also T. A. Shannon and J. J. Walter, "The PVS Patient and the Forgoing/ Withdrawing of Medical Nutrition and Hydration," in *Quality of Life*, pp. 203–23.

28. Congregation for the Doctrine of the Faith, "Declaration on Euthanasia," in *Quality of Life*, pp. 259–64.

29. McCormick and Paris, "The Catholic Tradition on the Use of Nutrition and Fluids," p. 358. Two other Catholic reports on the moral responsibility in prolonging life decisions not noted above have been advanced by pontifical agencies. First, the Pontifical Council Cor Unum issued a report in 1981 dealing with the ethical aspects of providing medical care to person at the end-of-life (Pontifical Council Cor Unum. "Questions of Ethics Regarding the Fatally Ill and the Dying," in *Conserving Human Life*, 286–304). Second, the Pontifical Academy of Sciences issued a report in 1985 dealing with the moral obligation to use life-sustaining medical treatment and the criteria necessary for determining the exact moment of death (Pontifical Academy of Sciences, "The Artificial Prolongation of Life, and Exact Determination of the Moment of Death," in *Conserving Human Life*, 305–7). These reports seem to indicate that medically assisted nutrition and hydration should be considered "ordinary or proportionate" means of prolonging life and thus should be used unless death is imminent or they impose an excessive burden on the patient, but they lack the authoritative doctrinal status of papal teaching and statements of the Congregations. These reports were actually made *to* the pope, but they have not been "officially promulgated by him to date or made part of authoritative teaching" (Albert S. Moraczewski, "The Moral Opposition Not to Conserve Life Under Certain Conditions," in *Conserving Human Life*, 233–75, at 240).

30. See New Jersey Catholic Conference, "Providing Food and Fluids to Severely Brain Damaged Patients," *Origins* 16 (22 January 1987): 582–84.

31. See Texas Catholic Bishops and the Texas Conference of Catholic Health Facilities, "On Withdrawing Artificial Nutrition and Hydration," *Origins* 20 (7 June 1990): 53–55. This statement was signed by sixteen bishops, with two bishops declining to sign.

32. See United States Bishops' Committee for Pro-Life Activities, "Nutrition and Hydration: Moral and Pastoral Reflections," *Origins* 21 (9 April 1992): 705–12.

33. Moraczewski, "The Moral Option Not to Conserve Life Under Certain Conditions," in *Conserving Human Life*, p. 243.

34. Second Vatican Council, *Gaudium et Spes*, n. 19, in *Proclaiming Justice and Peace: Papal Documents from Rerum Novarum to Centesimus Annus*, rev. and exp., ed. M. Walsh and B. Davies (Mystic, Conn.: Twenty-Third Publications, 1994), p. 169.

35. D. Brodeur, "Feeding Policy Protects Patients' Rights, Decisions," *Health Progress* (June 1985): 38–43, at 39.

36. Walter, "The Meaning and Validity of Quality of Life Judgments in Contemporary Roman Catholic Medical Ethics," in *Quality of Life*, pp. 85–86.

37. Pius XII, "The Prolongation of Life," in *Critical Choices and Critical Care*, 192. Orville Griese contends that this interpretation of Pius XII's statement is not correct insofar as it applies to removing medically assisted nutrition and hydration from dying patients ("Feeding the Hopeless and the Helpless," in *Conserving Human Life*, 147–232, at 157–58). Griese's main reason for

making this contention is that medically assisted nutrition and hydration is not medical treatment, as is mechanical ventilation, which is what Pius XII was specifically referring to in his reflections on the prolongation of life.

38. R. A. McCormick, "To Save or Let Die," in *Quality of Life*, pp. 26–34, at 30–31; B. Ashley and K. D. O'Rourke, *Health Care Ethics: A Theological Analysis*, 4th ed. (Washington, D.C.: Georgetown University Press, 1997), 424–26; Atkinson, *Pope Pius XII Speaks, The Prolongation of Life*, 9; Brodeur, "Feeding Policy Protects Patients' Rights, Decisions," p. 39; and K. D. O'Rourke and J. deBlois, "Removing Life Support: Motivations, Obligations," *Health Progress* 73 (July–August 1992): 20–27, at 24.

39. Ashley and O'Rourke, *Health Care Ethics*, 424–26; Atkinson, *Pope Pius XII Speaks: The Prolongation of Life*, 9; Brodeur, "Feeding Policy Protects Patients' Rights, Decisions," p. 39; and O'Rourke and deBlois, "Removing Life Support," p. 24.

40. R. McCormick, *How Brave a New World: Dilemmas in Bioethics* (Washington, D.C.: Georgetown University Press, 1981), p. 350.

41. The primary architect of the incommensurable or basic goods theory is Germain Grisez who first laid out the fundamental dimensions of this theory in an early work entitled *Contraception and the Natural Law* (Milwaukee: Bruce, 1964). Grisez later expanded the theory in a book coauthored with J. M. Boyle, B. Cole, J. M. Finnis, J. A. Geinzer, J. Grisez, R. G. Kennedy, P. Lee, W. E. May, and R. Shaw, *The Way of the Lord Jesus*, vol. 1: *Christian Moral Principles* (Chicago: Franciscan Herald Press, 1983). W. E. May has provided an accessible account of Grisez's approach in *Becoming Human* (Dayton: Pflaum, 1975); and *An Introduction to Moral Theology* (Huntington, Ind.: Our Sunday Visitor Press, 1991). The incommensurable or basic goods theory has received its most substantial presentation from J. Finnis in two of his books, namely: *Fundamentals of Ethics* (Washington, D.C.: Georgetown University Press, 1983); and *Natural Law and Natural Rights* (Oxford: Clarendon Press, 1984).

42. Finnis *Fundamentals of Ethics*, p. 51; and *Natural Law and Natural Rights*, pp. 85–90.

43. K. O'Rourke, "On the Care of 'Vegetative' Patients: A Response to William E. May's 'Tube Feeding and the Vegetative State': Part Two," *Ethics and Medics* 24 (May 1999): 3–4. at 3. Some of the authors who either explicitly or implicitly espouse the incommensurable or basic goods theory seem to arrive at this conclusion. See, for instance, R. Barry, *Medical Ethics: Essays on Abortion and Euthanasia* (New York: Peter Lang, 1989), 179–200 and 236–62; G. Grisez, et al., *The Way of the Lord Jesus*, pp. 214–225; and W. E. May, "Tube Feeding and the 'Vegetative' State: Part One," *Ethics and Medics* 23 (December 1998): 1–2.

44. Congregation for the Doctrine of the Faith, "Declaration on Euthanasia," in *Quality of Life*, p. 263.

45. Moraczewski, "The Moral Option Not to Conserve Life Under Certain Conditions," in *Conserving Human Life*, p 255.

46. Walter discusses the notion of benefit as understood in the Catholic tradition in "The Meaning and Validity of Quality of Life Judgments in Contemporary Roman Catholic Medical Ethics," in *Quality of Life*, pp. 85–86. Walter points out that "when medicine can intervene to ameliorate the quality of the relation between the patient's condition and the pursuit of life's goals, then such an intervention can be considered a benefit to the patient and is in his/her best interests" (p. 85).

47. W. H. Bullock, "Assessing Burdens and Benefits of Medical Care," *Origins* 21 (30 January 1992): 553–55, at 554.

48. See B. M. Ashley, "Contemporary Understanding of Personhood," in *The Twenty-Fifth Anniversary of Vatican II: A Look Back and A Look Ahead* (Braintree, Mass.: Pope John Center, 1990), 35–48; C. G. Brunk, "In the Image of God," in *Medical Ethics, Human Choices: A Christian Perspective*, ed. J. Rogers (Scottsdale, Penn.: Herald Press, 1988), pp. 29–40; R. M. Gula, *Reason Informed by Faith: Foundations of Catholic Morality* (New York: Paulist Press, 1989), pp. 66–74; L. Janssens, "Personalist Morals," *Louvain Studies* 3 (Spring 1970): 5–16; J. B. Reichmann, *Philosophy of the Human Person* (Chicago: Loyola University Press, 1985), pp. 207–25.

49. W. E. May, R. L. Barry, O. N. Griese, G. Grisez, B. V. Johnstone, T. J. Marzen, J. T. McHugh, G. Meilaender, M. Siegler, and W. B. Smith, "Feeding and Hydrating the Permanently Unconscious and Other Vulnerable Persons," in *Quality of Life*, 195–202, at 200. May does not say as much, but it is clear that his concept of benefit presupposes that human life is a good that cannot be weighted against other goods. If so, the criticisms of the theory of incommensurable goods apply also to May's argument.

50. R. A. McCormick, *Corrective Vision: Explorations in Moral Theology* (Kansas City: Sheed and Ward, 1994), p. 232.

51. Moraczewski, "The Moral Option Not to Conserve Life Under Certain Conditions," in *Conserving Human Life*, p. 257. Most Catholic theologians concur that medically assisted nutrition and hydration is a medical treatment and is subject to the same moral standards as other treatments. See Brodeur, "Feeding Policy Protects Patients' Rights, Decisions," p. 43; R. A. McCormick, *The Critical Calling: Reflections on Moral Dilemmas Since Vatican II* (Washington, D.C.: Georgetown University Press, 1989), pp. 380–81; and see O'Rourke and deBlois, "Removing Life Support: Motivations, Obligations," p. 25.

52. See B. M. Ashley, "Ethical Obligations," in *Scarce Medical Resources and Justice* (Braintree, Mass.: Pope John Center, 1987), 159–65, at 161; See O'Rourke, "On the Care of 'Vegetative' Patients: A Response to William E. May's 'Tube Feeding and the Vegetative State': Part One," p. 3; P. A. Talone, *Feeding the Dying: Religion and End-of-Life Decisions* (New York: Peter Lang, 1996), p. 21.

53. Cronin, *Conserving Human Life*, p. 88; See ref. 29, Moraczewski, "The Moral Option Not to Conserve Life Under Certain Conditions," in *Conserving Human Life*, pp. 261–62.

54. Moraczewski, "The Moral Option Not to Conserve Life Under Certain Conditions," in *Conserving Human Life*, p. 264. For a discussion of how to deal with the emotional responses of patients, family members, and medical professionals in decisions to withdraw life-sustaining medical treatment, see G. Povar, "Withdrawing and Withholding Therapy: Putting Ethics into Practice," *Journal of Clinical Ethics* 1 (Spring 1990): 50–56.

4

A History of Ordinary and Extraordinary Means

Donald E. Henke

The death of Terri Schiavo in Florida on March 31, 2005, brought into high relief many of the central questions concerning the care and treatment of patients
in the persistent vegetative state (PVS). At the center of the Catholic discussion of this contentious issue has been whether the provision of food and water
is an extraordinary means of conserving life when a patient no longer has any
measurable cognitive-affective abilities. Although my own work on the topic of
artificially assisted hydration and nutrition (AAHN) is involved with the question of whether such patients are indeed incapable of awareness of themselves
and others, that issue is not addressed here.[1] This article will consider the topic
of ordinary and extraordinary means as the background for the larger discussion
within the Church over the appropriate care of PVS patients. After a survey of
key historical ideas in the development of this distinction, I conclude with some
comments on how the distinction between ordinary and extraordinary treatment
helped the bishops and the Church's magisterium to arrive at the conclusion that
the provision of food and water is morally obligatory, in most cases, for those
who are in the PVS.

Ordinary and Extraordinary Means of Preserving Life

Catholic teaching regarding human life starts from more general principles that
delineate the ultimate nature of the human person, and then moves to more

specific principles aimed at safeguarding human dignity and caring for human life within the bounds of health care. Because human life is a precious gift of God, the positive requirements incumbent upon the human person demand that he assume a reasonable degree of care for his life; however, because human life is not an absolute good to be maintained at all costs, there are equally important limits to this duty. The efforts of the Church throughout its history to outline the duty and limits of caring for human life has resulted in a solid moral tradition that advocates the use of all ordinary means to preserve life, along with a right to forgo any extraordinary means to preserve life.

The vitally important address by Pope Pius XII in 1957 to a group of Catholic physicians and anesthesiologists gave a succinct statement of the Church's position regarding the ordinary and extraordinary means of conserving life. The Pope stated:

> Normally one is held to use only ordinary means—according to circumstances of persons, places, times, and culture—that is to say, means that do not involve any grave burden for oneself or another. A more strict obligation would be too burdensome for most men and would render the attainment of the higher, more important good too difficult. Life, health, all temporal activities, are in fact subordinated to spiritual ends. On the other hand, one is not forbidden to take more than the strictly necessary steps to preserve life and health, as long as he does not fail in some more serious duty.[2]

In 1958, the theological study by Daniel Cronin constructed a comprehensive analysis of the Church's moral tradition pertaining to the ordinary and extraordinary means of conserving human life.[3] The treatment of this subject in my article will present a representative selection of the theologians who clarified the major tenets of the obligations and limits correlative to the preservation of life. The brief examination of the principles governing the care of human life will provide both a glimpse into the course of historical development of the Catholic moral tradition and an important reference point for the arguments used to promote the provision or withholding of AAHN to the PVS patient, which will be discussed later.

Historical Roots and Use of the Terms

In the course of his research, Cronin discovered that the seeds upon which the ordinary and extraordinary means of preserving life would later grow were to be found in the treatises of St. Thomas Aquinas, particularly in his treatment of suicide and bodily mutilation.[4] Of significant value for later theologians, who more thoroughly addressed the demands and limits of a human person's responsibility to preserve his life, was this statement of St. Thomas: "A man has the obligation to sustain his body, otherwise he would be a killer of himself . . . by precept, therefore, he is bound to nourish his body and likewise, we are bound to all the other items without which the body cannot live."[5]

While this statement did not specifically delineate the precise elements that make up the obligation to preserve life, or even mention the instances and circumstances which would limit this duty, it did clearly maintain that the responsibility to preserve human life does exist and that it is a serious obligation, or else a person "would be a killer of himself." St. Thomas's broad statement on the somewhat tangential issue of suicide could be regarded as the kernel of what would become a significant moral study on the care of human life. From this point forward, as human needs have demanded, other theologians have built upon, and slowly developed, more specific duties and limits to the obligation noted by St. Thomas.

The theologians of the sixteenth century, especially Francisco de Vitoria (d. 1546) and Dominic Soto, O.P. (d. 1560), provided the next advances in the moral growth of the specific requirements to preserve human life. In Cronin's assessment, the contribution of Vitoria involved the specific obligation of the human person to eat food and thus sustain life, which Vitoria based primarily upon the human person's natural inclination to self-conservation.[6] Of equal importance to the positive requirement of taking food to preserve life were the limits he placed upon that obligation:

> Thirdly, I would say that if the depression of spirit is so low and there is present such consternation in the appetitive power that only with the greatest of effort and as though by means of a certain torture, can the sick man take food, right away that is reckoned in a certain impossibility, and therefore he is excused, at least from mortal sin, especially where there is little hope of life, or none at all.[7]

In this paragraph, Vitoria demonstrated an understanding that the duty to preserve life by taking food was not an absolute obligation, and, in so doing, he established the rudimentary threads that acknowledged the existence of circumstances where impossibility or extreme difficulty interfered with compliance with the positive obligation of conserving life. Other factors delineated by Vitoria that mitigated the duty to preserve life have been noted by John Connery,

SJ, who states, "one is not obliged to use foods which are the best, the most expensive or the most exquisite. Neither is one bound to live in the healthiest climate . . . those who refuse to take some particular medicine are not to be condemned since one can rarely be certain that it will work."[8] One can notice, therefore, that the scope of the obligation to conserve life is fixed at reasonable measures, with common foods, in normal settings, and with medicines that are known to be effective.

Dominic Soto, OP, offered little in the way of innovation in any sense that built upon Aquinas and Vitoria, but he was the first to address some of the duties and limits pertaining to surgery, in particular those surrounding acceptance of amputation. Connery notes that Soto asks "whether one is bound to undergo amputation of an arm or leg to preserve or prolong life. His answer is that no one could force a patient to undergo such torture."[9] Before the advent of reliable anesthetics, the question of what could reasonably be asked of a patient in terms of mutilation or amputation was frequently discussed, and the common opinion concluded that such a course was usually beyond the level required to preserve life, because of the great pain involved.[10] Regarding the pain of overbearing shame, both Leonardus Lessius and Gabriel of St. Vincent concurred that an experience of excessive shame or abhorrence related to a medical procedure could also be more than a person should be asked to bear, and thus a reasonable cause to forgo the treatment. In this instance, both theologians were specifically referring to the care of female patients by male physicians.[11]

Juan Cardinal de Lugo (d. 1660) provided the next significant addition to the moral tradition regarding ordinary and extraordinary means of conserving life. The moral theology of de Lugo offered several nuances that were not so much highly innovative as they were subtle insights and clarifications serving to broaden the Catholic moral tradition regarding the lengths and limits of conserving life. A particularly interesting contribution found in de Lugo's moral theology involved a deeper understanding of extraordinary means. Instead of automatically accepting the extraordinary status of an amputation, a procedure that would likely save a person's life but would entail intense pain, de Lugo took a different tack. Thomas O'Donnell, SJ, remarked that "De Lugo himself does not presuppose the extraordinary difficulty of a leg amputation, as [Saint Alphonsus Liguori] seems to do."[12] De Lugo stated, "He must permit this cure when the doctors judge it necessary, and when it can happen without intense pain; not, if it is accompanied by very bitter pain; because a man is not bound to employ extraordinary and difficult means to conserve his life."[13]

In this statement, de Lugo shrewdly observed that the difficulty presented in the amputation procedure lay primarily with the significant amount of pain that often accompanied it and not necessarily with the amputation procedure itself. Hence, the extraordinary nature of an amputation, de Lugo realized, lay in the overwhelming pain, and not necessarily in the amputation itself. In a case in which the obscuring blanket of pain was removed, the amputation procedure could constitute an ordinary means of conserving life.

A second vital contribution which Cardinal de Lugo provided for the Catholic moral tradition was a greater clarification of the distinction between the positive formulation of the obligations necessary to preserve life (namely, the ordinary means of preserving life) and the negative formulation of the actions a person was not required to perform in order to preserve his life (namely, the extraordinary means of preserving life). Cronin's assessment of de Lugo showed the latter's firm conviction that the positive requirements to preserve the great good of human life using ordinary means were absolutely necessary, and a refusal to use them was the moral equivalent to suicide. De Lugo made his conviction clear in the following paragraph:

> [A] man must guard his life by ordinary means against dangers and death coming from natural causes . . . because the one who neglects the ordinary means seems to neglect his life and therefore to act negligently in the administration of it, and he who does not employ the ordinary means which nature has provided for the ordinary conservation of life is considered morally to will his death.[14]

De Lugo then examined the limits of the human person's responsibility to conserve his life. He offered a clear distinction between the death of a person because of inadequate use of the ordinary means (which was a moral violation) and the death of a person resulting from a decision not to use an extraordinary means (which was not a moral violation). De Lugo reasoned that a human person's life was not the greatest good, namely, something to be preserved at all costs; hence, a decision to only use ordinary means is morally acceptable. He stated that one

> is not held to the extraordinary and difficult means . . . the "bonum" of his life is not of such great moment . . . that its conservation must be effected with extraordinary diligence: it is one thing not to neglect and rashly throw it away, to which a man is bound: it is another, however, to seek after it and retain it by exquisite means as it is escaping away from him, to which he is not held; neither is he on that account considered morally to will or seek his death.[15]

His analysis of the extraordinary means considered the various options available to prolong one's life, ranging from the use of expensive foods and medicines to the taking or abstaining from wine,[16] all of which he deemed not morally obligatory.

In the midst of this treatment of the extraordinary means, however, a third important contribution of de Lugo emerged. He introduced the concept of proportional benefit, in which, within the domain of an ordinary means of preserving life, circumstances could exist which effectively rendered such a means extraordinary. Using the example of a man surrounded by fire and facing certain death by that fire, de Lugo illustrated the concept of proportional benefit.[17] The man in the fire has at hand, in de Lugo's scenario, enough water to extinguish part of the fire, but not all of it, and if he used the water to quench some of the fire, his certain death would be delayed only a short time. In this case, the crucial element that determines proportional benefit is whether there exists a reasonable hope of recovery or continued life for an extended period of time, not simply a few extra moments. Ultimately, de Lugo reasoned that if a proposed action, medicine, or food, even if ordinary in itself, provided no significant assistance to the preservation of life, i.e., no proportional benefit, such a means was extraordinary and, therefore, nonobligatory. In short, the principle that emerged from this new theological insight was one that would have significant ramifications for moralists who later assessed the proportional benefit of providing AAHN to PVS patients: namely, that no one was obligated to employ a useless means.[18]

The next addition which honed the Catholic moral tradition regarding ordinary and extraordinary means involved an assessment regarding the level of pain required before a means became extraordinary. The seventeenth century theologian H. Tournely posed the question of the person who did not want to undergo treatment that entailed suffering even moderate pain to conserve his life, and asked if such an individual could be forced to undergo such treatment. He responded, as later theologians also did, that a treatment involving extreme pain did not impose an obligation on a person. However, a person did have the duty to accept a proposed treatment offering only moderate pain, and he could be forced to submit to it by those caring for him. Tournely concluded that the suffering of moderate pain with such treatment did not contain a moral impossibility, and thus it would constitute an obligatory means to conserve a person's life.[19] This determination would be particularly useful in the modern health-care arena, in which the availability of effective anesthetics can reduce nearly all pain to manageable levels.

By the middle of the nineteenth century, speculation began regarding the use of induced sleep to relieve the intense pain of amputations and other surgeries. John Gury and other theologians questioned the obligation of a person to accept an operation if the experience of pain would be absent due to some form of artificially induced sleep. While the advent of anesthesia would provide the benefit of eliminating or greatly reducing the pain associated with medical treatments of this type, Gury ultimately concluded that the unknown dangers of an induced sleep, the loss of reason for an extended period of time, and the overall uncertainty of the sleep-inducing procedure made it an extraordinary means of conserving life.[20] The use and reliability of anesthetics aside, late-nineteenth-century theologians also considered the major surgery of amputation likely to constitute an extraordinary means, because of the difficulty inherent in living with its after-effects, i.e., subjective repugnance, in addition to the surgery itself. Gerald Kelly quotes Palmieri, who said:

> Theologians are speaking of the intense pains of amputation. But what if the use of an anesthetic removes the pain? Could we not still say that the serious inconvenience of living with a mutilated body would just as readily excuse the patient from undergoing the amputation as would the very intense pains that last only a short time?[21]

The hesitancy among early-twentieth-century moral theologians to acknowledge the effectiveness and reliability of anesthetics slowly gave way to a gradual acceptance of their advantages, largely through the efforts of Dr. C. Capellmann, who promoted the advances of medical science at that time and applied the tenets of moral theology to them.[22] The result was that the status of certain operations like amputation, which nearly always were accorded extraordinary status due to pain or difficulty, became less automatically pronounced as such. The theological assessment of H. Noldin and A. Schmitt in 1941 illustrated this modification in thought:

> Today the suffering is vastly decreased through narcotics, the danger of infection is very remote, and moreover success is more frequent and assured, and even for amputated members, there are artificial limbs—and therefore, at least where certain danger of death would very probably be avoided through an operation, it

does not seem that it can be called an extraordinary means, unless there is great subjective horror of it.[23]

Up to this point, the general consensus of moral theologians was that "man is obliged to take the ordinary means to preserve his life but is not obliged to use extraordinary means unless some demand of the common good enters into the picture. All agreed that means which would involve extreme pain, significant danger of death, excessive expense, or great subjective repugnance were to be classified as extraordinary."[24]

However, by the middle of the twentieth century, the rapid growth of available treatments in the medical field, the advent of more readily obtainable medicines, and improved medical facilities brought about a transformation in the character of health care. Of particular note were the advances made through use of artificial life-support technology. Modern medical techniques required theologians to speculate on the new moral questions raised by advanced medical technology as well as on the increasing complexity their use caused for the determination of ordinary and extraordinary means of conserving life.

Gerald Kelly, SJ, in his timely 1950 article, "The Duty of Using Artificial Means of Preserving Life," drew attention to the critical issues and questions posed by modern medical advances, with specific emphasis on artificial life-sustaining technology and the impact it had on the ordinary and extraordinary means of conserving human life. Interestingly, Kelly's assessment of the challenges confronting moral theology by 1950s medical care could, with a few additions, easily be reiterated today. He commented:

Our age abounds in artificial means of preserving life: e.g., incubators, blood transfusion, oxygen tents and masks, iron lungs, highly technical operations, insulin, and various other stimulants and medications. The formulation of some definite rules concerning the duty of using these artificial means is not merely intriguing speculation; it is also—if I may judge from the many questions asked me—a practical necessity.[25]

Moral theologians in the latter half of the twentieth century have been faced with the daunting task of applying the Catholic moral tradition regarding the preservation of human life within the context of the many stunning advances in medical technology, particularly the provision of artificial life support. In a few instances, notably in the early part of the twentieth century, a position had been put forward which stipulated that anything not natural was automatically extraordinary, and therefore a nonobligatory means of conserving human life.[26] This determination, however, seemed to be somewhat simplistic given the ease of obtaining and using some artificially produced medicines and procedures. O'Donnell commented that

> It would lead to a position wherein the modern antibiotics, by the mere fact that they are artificially produced and administered, would be considered extraordinary means of preserving life. Moreover, although we must note and remember for future consideration that there is a valid distinction between natural and artificial means, still the artificial is not to be considered as wholly distinct from the natural. The advances of modern science are due fundamentally to the development of the natural potentialities of civilized man living in society, with each generation building on the discoveries and achievements of the last, as is evidently in accord with the rational nature of man. Thus it is inauspicious to say that surgery, intravenous feeding, radiation therapy, and the like, are extraordinary means, because they are, in themselves, artificial and unnatural. They are not properly considered in themselves, but rather must be viewed in their historical context.[27]

Kelly supported a proposal that classified all artificial means of sustaining life as a remedy for a particular disease or illness. The distinguishing characteristic of a remedy was that an individual might employ it as a useful means toward recovering from or halting a disease. However, a person incurred no obligation to use a remedy unless it offered a "reasonable hope of success" pertaining to the cure or alleviation of some aspect of a disease.[28] The example he used was a person breathing with supplemental oxygen. He remarked that "It is one thing to use oxygen to bring a person through a crisis; it is another thing to use it merely to prolong life when hope for recovery is practically negligible."[29] The heart of Kelly's position pertaining to artificial means of preserving life concluded that, based upon a "prudent, human evaluation," the degree to which a particular means cured or controlled a disease determined whether it was ordinary or extraordinary. Simply because a means to preserve life was not completely natural did not mean that it automatically became extraordinary.[30] Cronin agreed. He remarked that, "the terms artificial means and extraordinary means are not coextensive. An artificial means can be an ordinary means of conserving life?"[31]

To conclude this brief historical overview, it can be noted that Gerald Kelly provided a helpful definition of the ordinary and extraordinary means of conserving life. His definition formulated the ordinary and extraordinary means in such a way that each was completely exclusive from the other. Atkinson summarized Kelly, saying,

> In other words, to call a means nonobligatory one must, using Kelly's new definitions, call the means extraordinary. Ordinary = obligatory, extraordinary = per se optional, and these two equations are justified by reducing the obligatoriness of means to their being easily obtained and employed and their offering reasonable hope of benefit.[32]

In this way, Kelly sought to reduce ambiguities that might affect the practical application of it in a moral determination. For him, the ordinary and extraordinary means were best defined in the following way:

> *Ordinary* means are all medicines, treatments, and operations, which offer a reasonable hope of benefit and which can be obtained and used without excessive expense, pain, or other inconvenience.
>
> *Extraordinary* means are all medicines, treatments and operations, which cannot be obtained or used without excessive expense, pain, or other inconvenience, or which, if used, would not offer a reasonable hope of benefit.[33]

These definitions were the result of the four-hundred-year tradition of the Church, and at the same time, they possessed the capacity to assess the techniques and treatments of modern medicine.

Clarifying the Ordinary and Extraordinary Means

The work of Cronin further sharpened the distinction between ordinary and extraordinary means of conserving life and even more completely illustrated the importance of the individual in his fullness (i.e., to include physical condition, mental and emotional state, etc.) as the integral cog in these determinations. In assessing Kelly's definitions, Cronin concluded that they seemed too focused upon clinical procedures, and thus were not broad enough to include other means of conserving life. In Cronin's estimation, it was also incumbent upon a comprehensive definition to include the concept of reasonable difficulty when weighing ordinary means, thereby demonstrating the belief that while a moral impossibility makes a particular action extraordinary, a reasonable difficulty did not. Finally, the addition of the other major elements that make up ordinary and extraordinary means enabled him to formulate the following definitions:

Ordinary means of conserving life are those means commonly used in given circumstances, which this individual in his present physical, psychological and economic condition can reasonably employ with definite hope of proportional benefit.

Extraordinary means of conserving life are those means not commonly used in given circumstances, or those means in common use which this individual in his present physical, psychological and economic condition cannot reasonably employ, or if he can, will not give him definite hope of proportionate benefit.[34]

Cronin was quick to point out that these definitions were not absolute norms.[35] Accordingly, the individual person was the only one with the ability to accurately assess the benefits or burdens of a particular means, for the simple reason that each person experienced the effects of a particular treatment, operation, or medicine differently. What might be an ordinary means of conserving life for one person could be extraordinary for someone else. Kelly noticed this problem earlier when he remarked that:

The foregoing definitions do not avoid all difficulties. There is always difficulty in estimating such factors as "excessive," "reasonable hope," "proportional benefit," and so forth. But this difficulty seems inherent in all attempts to make human estimates, and it is doubtful that we can ever attain to a formulation that will entirely remove this problem.[36]

Cronin did, however, examine each of the essential elements of the ordinary and extraordinary means of conserving life, to clarify the terms as sharply as possible.

Within the domain of the ordinary means of conserving human life, Cronin delineated five categories that made a particular aspect of health care or medical treatment ordinary and therefore obligatory: [37]

1. Hope of a beneficial result *(spes salutis)*: The heart of this requirement was that any means to conserve life, whether natural or artificial, even common means like food and water must offer a proportional benefit for those means to acquire obligatory status. This benefit, based on the observations of de Lugo (i.e., the analogy of the man condemned to fire) "must be worthwhile in quality and duration. Furthermore, it must be worthwhile in consideration of the effort expended in using the means."[38]

2. Common use of means *(media communia)*: Nearly all moral theologians from Vitoria to the present referred in one way or another to the requirement that the means used to conserve life be common. This stipulation

applied to all aspects of care, ranging from food to medicine to living conditions, even to the level of attention one gave to the preservation of his or her life. The care one owed to the preservation of human life did not extend beyond normal conscientious observance. The relative nature of determining what precisely constituted "common" in this sense was based upon the subsequent pillar of the ordinary means.

3. According to social position (*secundum proportionem status*): The factor of social status was intended to indicate the available economic resources possessed by a particular patient, which could heavily affect the idea of what precisely "common" would comprise for such an individual. There were limits, however, to what even wealthy people would be required to do to preserve their lives.[39]

4. Means not too difficult to obtain or use (*media non difficilia*): The conclusion reached by moral theologians determined that the operative concept here was that the means could not be excessively difficult to obtain if a person were to remain obligated to employ them. "They clearly state, however, that a moderate difficulty does not constitute an extraordinary means. Furthermore, from a study of their writings, one cannot say that the moralists teach that the terms "difficulty" and "ordinary means" are mutually exclusive."[40] This caveat applied to the acquisition of necessary foods and medicines, and also to enduring pain and the risk of the treatment, to name a few.

5. Means are easy to obtain or use (*media facilia*): Closely connected to, but less often used by moral theologians than *media non difficilia*, was the concept of *media facilia*. At its heart, the term signified that the means employed by an individual to conserve his or her life should be able to be obtained or used with a reasonable amount of convenience. Cronin pointed out that this did not imply that no difficulty whatsoever should be involved in using such means, but that the term "reasonable" was closer to the intended meaning of the phrase "easy to obtain or use."[41]

The elements gleaned from the Catholic moral tradition regarding the extraordinary means of conserving life were likewise categorized by Cronin into five major areas:[42]

I. Certain impossibility (*quaedam impossibilitas*): The theological principle used by Cronin and other moral theologians was based upon the understanding that one was not always required to do a positive good; in this case, the human person was not always bound to conserve his life at all costs. Hence, the presence of a moral or physical impossibility, namely, a difficulty of sufficient magnitude to warrant a nonobligatory status relative to the condition of the patient, was enough to classify the difficulty as an extraordinary means of conserving life. In this instance, as with the other elements that made up the ordinary and extraordinary means of conserving life, the crucial decision must lie with the person experiencing the difficulty.[43]

2. Great effort or too difficult *(summus labor* and *media nimis dura):* This guideline affirmed that while a person was obligated to expend reasonable levels of effort in the preservation of his life, any effort that extended beyond the level of reasonable to the excessive would be classified as extraordinary.

3. Unbearable suffering and pain *(quidam cruciatus* and *ingens dolor):* The intense experience of pain and suffering, relative to the condition of the individual person, was nearly always cited as grounds to declare a particular treatment, operation, or type of care a moral impossibility. While the introduction of anesthetics has lessened the overwhelming presence of pain in the present age, the presence of pain and suffering remains a significant factor that must be assessed on a person-by-person basis.

4. Unreasonable expense *(sumptus extraordinarius, media pretiosa,* and *media exquisita):* According to an individual's social status or financial well-being, the issue of excessive expense, relatively calculated, has been advanced by centuries of moralists as an extraordinary means.

5. Unreasoning fear or repugnance *(vehemens horror):* The final category that denoted a moral impossibility pertained to instances in which a particular medical action produced intense levels of fear or disgust in the mind and heart of a patient. Under the circumstances in which a particular individual was so completely overcome with fear or repugnance, a procedure of this nature could become extraordinary.[44]

Further Developments Regarding the Ordinary and Extraordinary Means

The conclusion of the overview of the ordinary and extraordinary means of conserving life, specifically as it pertains to the PVS patient, is not complete without a momentary look at two major developments that have sprung from it. The first development within the tradition of the ordinary and extraordinary means came from the address by Pope Pius XII on the moral implications of prolonging life. In his remarks, mentioned above, the Pope directly addressed the obligations of a person to conserve his life. Because of its importance, his statement is worth repeating here:

> Normally one is held to use only ordinary means—according to circumstances of persons, places, times, and culture—that is to say, means that do not involve any grave burden for oneself or another. A more strict obligation would be too burdensome for most men and would render the attainment of the higher, more important good too difficult. Life, health, all temporal activities, are in fact subordinated to spiritual ends. On the other hand, one is not forbidden to take more than the strictly necessary steps to preserve life and health, as long as he does not fail in some more serious duty.[45]

This statement—in particular, the Pope's mention of "the attainment of the higher, more important good" and the subordination of life to "spiritual ends"—became a focal point from which theologians argued the extraordinary, and therefore non-obligatory, character of providing AAHN to patients in conditions diagnosed as PVS.[46] Kevin O'Rourke, OP, held this position and stated:

> Pope Pius XII, when speaking about life support systems, declared: "Life, health, all temporal activities are in fact subordinated to spiritual ends." Thus, when the potential for spiritual function is no longer present, then it seems that all treatment or care efforts which would sustain physiological function are ineffective.[47]

The second important development within the Catholic moral tradition of the ordinary and extraordinary means of conserving life occurred due to confusion arising from the manner in which the health-care community used the terms, in contrast to the traditional theological meaning of the terms. Bryan Jennett's understanding of the ordinary and extraordinary means of conserving life highlighted the difficulty between the medical and theological confusion. He commented:

> Since the Pope's 1957 declaration that physicians are normally obliged to use only ordinary means to preserve life, there have been debates about how to distinguish these from extraordinary treatments. Initially ordinary was taken to mean generally available and widely used, whilst extraordinary would include advanced technological methods that were scarce and expensive.[48]

In an attempt to clarify the distinction between what the medical community understood as the definitional characteristics of the terms *ordinary* and
extraordinary, described by Jennett, and the theological understanding, which
was significantly more nuanced than simple ease or difficulty in application,
the Congregation for the Doctrine of the Faith (CDF) responded with its
1980 *Declaration on Euthanasia*. The declaration proposed that the terms used by
moral theologians and medical personnel should shift away from the *ordinary–
extraordinary* distinction, which had recently become a source of misunderstanding, to a different set of terms that would be more specific. The document
indicated that

> In the past moralists replied that one is never obliged to use "extraordinary"
> means. This reply, which as a principle still holds good, is perhaps less clear
> today by reason of the imprecision of the term and the rapid progress made in
> the treatment of sickness. Thus some people prefer to speak of "proportionate"
> and "disproportionate" means.
>
> In any case, it will be possible to make a correct judgment as to the means
> by studying the type of treatment to be used, its degree of complexity or risk,
> its cost and the possibilities of using it, and comparing these elements with the
> result that can be expected, taking into account the state of the sick person and
> his or her physical and moral resources [49]

In this way, the CDF offered the terms *proportionate* and *disproportionate* as a
substitute, to avoid the confusion that had crept into the application of the
terms *ordinary* and *extraordinary*. Instead of centering attention on the treatment
alone as common and inexpensive or technologically advanced and expensive, as
had been the practice within the medical community, the Catholic moral tradition pointed to more comprehensive guidelines. As O'Donnell indicated, the
terms *proportionate* and *disproportionate* were not intended to classify means according to "a consideration of the therapeutic measures considered in themselves,
but rather considered 'relatively' to the condition and circumstances of the individual patient."[50]

The Obligatory or Optional Classification of AAHN

Generally, every group concerned with health-care issues has agreed that the provision of basic nursing care was an aspect of medical care owed to all patients,

including the PVS patient. The universally accepted elements that constituted basic nursing care included simple actions or articles required to maintain personal hygiene and dignity; for example, proper clothing, temperature control, cleanliness, and even food and water for those who could consume them orally. Basic nursing care was considered, by all accounts, an aspect of medical care that should always be provided to patients regardless of the severity of their condition. Nevertheless, the specific characteristics of AAHN made it difficult to determine whether it should be classified as an aspect of normal care or as a medical treatment. Because the purpose of AAHN was to deliver food and fluids, many ethicists, lawyers, and medical personnel concluded that it was simply an aspect of the normal care owed to any patient; however, others determined that the requirement of skilled medical professionals to administer AAHN necessarily made it a medical treatment. In the end, although some in the Catholic tradition maintained that the provision of AAHN was obligatory because it was an example of basic care, several documents issued under the umbrella of the Church hierarchy in America ultimately determined that the nature of AAHN was not the critical factor that made AAHN provision obligatory or optional.[51]

The Determination of Catholic Moral Theology Regarding AAHN

At the most basic level, the heart of the Catholic moral tradition regarding the proper care of the PVS patient has sought to determine whether AAHN was an ordinary (proportionate) means of preserving life, or whether it should be considered an extraordinary (disproportionate) means of preserving life. Thus, leaving aside the question of whether AAHN was believed to be an aspect of basic nursing care or a medical treatment, the fundamental reason why its provision was determined to be obligatory centered on the assessment that AAHN was an ordinary means of conserving life. For some Catholic organizations and theologians, the provision of food and water, whether delivered orally or through a feeding tube, was an aspect of basic nursing care on a par with hygienic measures, clothing, and proper temperature control.[52] Within this concept was the understanding that as long as food and water accomplished its intended purpose, namely, maintaining the life of the patient, it was an ordinary means of conserving life. Only under the specific circumstances in which a patient was imminently dying or the body could no longer assimilate nourishment would it become optional. Thus, to remove AAHN from a PVS patient whose life could be easily maintained by the provision of food and fluids was to withdraw an ordinary means of sustaining life and, as a consequence, to directly intend the death of the patient by dehydration.[53]

Later attempts of bishops' committees to address the issue of AAHN provision to PVS patients used a slightly different approach. Instead of resting their argument on the contention that AAHN was an example of basic care that must nearly always be provided to patients, these documents contended that the distinction between "treatments," which may be discontinued, and "care," which must be continued, did not offer a complete resolution to the problem, because both terms remained subject to the norms of ordinary and extraordinary means. Hence, as one document stated, "Whether it is viewed as treatment or care, it would be morally wrong to discontinue nutrition and hydration when they are within the realm of ordinary means."[54] From this later perspective, the key to determining whether the provision of AAHN to a PVS patient was morally obligatory or morally optional was to assess the benefits and burdens associated with its provision. The Pennsylvania bishops concluded that the provision of AAHN to PVS patients was clearly beneficial because it fulfilled the purpose for which it was given, namely, to sustain life. At the same time, the bishops determined that the provision of AAHN in these circumstances was not seriously burdensome, because it could be administered easily and with negligible amounts of pain or suffering.[55] Serious consideration was given to the charge that the excessive economic burdens of providing AAHN to a PVS patient made it an extraordinary means of preserving life; however, although these later documents acknowledged the serious financial burdens of caring for PVS patients, the U.S. Bishops' Pro-Life Committee believed that other options were available to make the cost of caring for PVS patients more manageable.[56] Both the Pennsylvania bishops and the U.S. Bishops' Pro-Life Committee advanced the belief that adequate assistance was available to make the provision of AAHN to PVS patients a financially affordable decision, especially in a society as affluent as the United States. The Pennsylvania bishops stated: "However, in the society in which we live this does not present a fully convincing argument. Resources are available from other sources, and these can often be tapped before a family reaches dire financial straits. Such assistance has been and continues to be available."[57]

It can be observed, therefore, that the Catholic moral stance regarding the decision to provide or withhold AAHN from PVS patients was based upon the criteria that are used to make the distinction between ordinary and extraordinary means of conserving life. The specific factors involved in the provision of AAHN to PVS patients led the majority of the American Catholic hierarchy to conclude that, based upon the current level of medical science, providing food and fluids to the PVS patient served a life-sustaining purpose that outweighed the minimal burdens that accompanied it, thus making it an ordinary means of conserving life that must be continued. While the distinction between the ordinary and extraordinary means of conserving life necessarily contained some subjective elements (the experience of excessive pain and suffering or financial concerns), not all of which were considered applicable to an irreversibly unconscious patient, the primary focus of the Catholic moral tradition was centered upon the benefit or burdensomeness of the particular treatment, in relation to the condition of the patient. In this manner, the Catholic moral tradition advocated an assessment process that took into consideration the specific circumstances of each patient, while at the same time holding to an objective decision-making framework. Thus, if a proposed treatment was deemed ordinary, there was a moral requirement to employ it; if a proposed treatment was deemed extraordinary, an option existed whether to apply it or not.

Although the publicly stated goal of both the Catholic Church and the American medical community regarding the care of patients is to provide effective medical care to treat a patient's injury or disease, it would seem that, in the case of the PVS patient, the decision of the Catholic Church to promote the provision of AAHN to sustain the patient's life is more in line with respect for the person than is a position that advocates the removal of AAHN so that the patient will die. In the end, because the evidence regarding the PVS patient's level of inner awareness is inconclusive, the decision to withhold or withdraw AAHN from a permanently unconscious patient comes too close to the abandonment of a person who cannot be cured. The position taken by the Catholic Church in relation to seriously ill patients has held that "the health-care worker who cannot affect a cure must never cease to treat."[58] Within the context of the PVS patient, the decision to treat through the delivery of AAHN is not an example of a vitalistic approach to health care that intends to maintain life at all costs. Rather, it is based on an assessment that the nondying patient can benefit from the provision of food and fluids that will sustain his life. At the same time, the AAHN given to the PVS patient is not determined to be excessively burdensome to receive, either in terms of pain, cost, or complexity. In the event that AAHN delivery was believed to be excessively burdensome for the

PVS patient, or if he could no longer assimilate the nutrients provided to him, it would probably no longer be an obligatory treatment.

The decision to provide AAHN to the PVS patient is ultimately grounded in an acceptance of the limitations placed upon the human person's autonomy by God, and compassion for a seriously debilitated patient who requires care. In the first place, it acknowledges that God is the master of life, and that even though existence in a PVS is perceived to be undesirable, the decision to remove AAHN to bring about the death of the patient lies outside the parameters for human action. Second, the decision to sustain the life of a PVS patient by providing AAHN involves a decision to recognize the value of a vulnerable patient's life and to remain in solidarity with him.[59] The true meaning of compassion, based upon love, involves maintaining contact with a suffering or seriously debilitated patient in the midst of his condition; compassion does not attempt to end the life of a patient because his continued existence is distressing. The decision to withhold or withdraw AAHN from PVS patients advances the belief that some lives are not worth preserving. In contrast, the decision to provide AAHN to PVS patients recognizes the incalculable worth of the human person and the intrinsic good of his life, regardless of his condition. In the end, the Catholic moral tradition considers no human life valueless.

Notes

1. For a consideration of this topic, see my thesis, *Artificially Assisted Nutrition and Hydration from Karen Quinlan to Nancy Cruzan to the Present: An Historical Analysis of the Decision to Provide or Withhold/Withdraw Sustenance from PVS Patients in Catholic Moral Theology and Medical Practice in the United States* (Rome: Pontificia Universitas Lateranensis–Academia Alfonsiana, 2004), esp. 41–66, "Regarding the PVS Patient."

2. Pius XII, "The Prolongation of Life: Allocution to the International Congress of Anesthesiologists" (November 24, 1957), *The Pope Speaks* 4.4 (1958): 395–98. While this statement by the Pope only addressed the broad strokes of the Church's position on the ordinary and extraordinary means of conserving life, it did have implications for the PVS patient. Some moral theologians, most notably Rev. Kevin D. O'Rourke, OP, used the statement of the Pope regarding "the attainment of the higher, more important good" to conclude that in the case of a permanently unconscious patient, hydration and nutrition could be forgone. This is discussed in a later section.

3. Daniel Cronin, *The Moral Law in Regard to the Ordinary and Extraordinary Means of Conserving Life* (Rome: Pontifical Gregorian University, 1958).

4. Cronin, *The Moral Law*, 47–48. Here, Cronin cites the commentary of Dominic Bañez on Thomas Aquinas (D. Bañez, *Scholastica Commentaria in Primam Partem Angelici Doctoris S. Thomae* [Duaci, 1614–1615], Tom. IV, Decisiones de Iure et Iustitia, in II: II. q. 65, art. 1).

5. Thomas Aquinas, *Super Epistolas S. Pauli* (Taurine-Romae: Marietti, 1953), II Thess., Lec. II, n. 77, in Cronin, *The Moral Law*, 48.

6. Cronin, *The Moral Law*, 48.

7. Francisco de Vitoria, *Relationes Theologiae* (Lugduni, 1587), Relectio IX. De temperantia, n. I, in Daniel Cronin, *The Moral Law*, 47–48.

8. Francisco de Vitoria, *Reflectiones Theologiae*, IX, De temperantia, n.I, in John Connery, SJ, "Prolonging Life: The Duty and Its Limits," *Linacre Quarterly* 47.2 (May 1980): 153. See also Francisco de Vitoria, *Commentarios a la Secunda Secundae de Santo Tomas* (ed. De Heredia, OP; Salamanca, 1952), in II: II, q. 147 art. I, cited in Daniel Cronin, *The Moral Law*, 50.

9. Connery, "Prolonging Life," 153; Connery quotes Dominic Soto, OP, *De Iustitia et Iure* (Venice 1568), Lib. 5, q. 2, a. I .

10. See Bañez, *Scholastica Commentaria in Primam partem Angelici Doctoris S. Thomae*, Tom. IV, Decisiones de Iure et Iustitia in II: II. q. 65, art I; L. Lessius, *De Iustitia et Iure* (Lugduni, 1622), Lib. II, Cap. 9, dub. 14, n. 96; Martin Bonacina, *Moralis Theologia* (Venetiis, 1721), Tom. II, disp. 2, quaest. Ultimo., sect. I punct. 6 n. 2; Paul Laymann, *Theologia Moralis* (Venetiis, 1719), Lib. III, Tract. III, p. 3, cap. I, n. 4.

11. L. Lessius, *De Iustitia et Iure*, Lib. IV, Cap.3, dub. 8, n. 60. He commented that "women, especially virgins, are not bound to accept from men medical treatment of this type in the more secret parts . . . The reason is because no one is held to accept a cure which he abhors no less than the disease itself or death." See also Gabrielis a St. Vincentio, *De Iustitia et Iure* (Rome: Mancini, 1663) disp. 6 de restitutione, q. 6, n. 86. Other theologians contradicted this position. See also Vincent Patuzzi, *Ethica Christiana sive Theologia Moralis* (Bassani, 1770), Tom. III, Tract. V, Pars. V, Cap. X, Consect. sept, cited in Gary M. Atkinson, "Theological History of Catholic Teaching on Prolonging Life," in *Moral Responsibility in Prolonging Life Decisions*, eds. Donald G. McCarthy and Albert S. Moraczewski, OP (St. Louis, MO: The Pope John XXIII Medical-Moral Research and Education Center, 1981), 104.

12. Thomas J. O'Donnell, SJ, *Medicine and Christian Morality*, 3rd ed. (NY: Alba House, 1996), 56. O'Donnell credited De Lugo for seeing past the barrier of intense pain from amputation to a future time when, due to proper anesthetics, pain would no longer be a significant factor in such a procedure. See also Atkinson, "Theological History of Catholic Teaching on Prolonging Life," 101. Atkinson commented that "the question at issue here is whether certain mutilations can become *obligatory*, as being necessary for life or health. De Lugo holds that such a mutilation is obligatory, *provided* that it can be accomplished without intense pain."

13. Juan Cardinal de Lugo, *Disputationes Scholasticae et Morales* (ed. Nova; Parisiis, Vivês, 1868–69), Vol. VI, De Iustitia et Iure, Disp. X, Sec. I n. 21.

14. Ibid., in Cronin, *The Moral Law*, 63.

15. Ibid., in Cronin, *The Moral Law*, 63–64.

16. Atkinson, "Theological History of Catholic Teaching on Prolonging Life," 101.

17. De Lugo, *Disputationes Scholasticae et Morales*, n. 30.

18. Connery, "Prolonging Life," 155. Richard A. McCormick, SJ, among other Catholic theologians, argued from this position regarding the provision of AAHN to PVS patients. In his book *The Critical Calling*, McCormick presented the reasoning of Daniel Callahan. McCormick remarked that "when all is said and done . . . Callahan allows cessation of nutrition-hydration for

those frail elderly who are 'imminently dying' and for those who are 'not dying but are irreversibly comatose, utterly vegetative.' For this latter category, nutrition and hydration simply confer no benefit. 'There is no meaningful life of any kind—it is a mere body only, not an embodied person. Thus there is nothing left that would deprive such a patient of something valuable.'" Richard A. McCormick, SJ, *The Critical Calling: Reflections on Moral Dilemmas since Vatican II* (Washington, DC: Georgetown University Press, 1989), 377.

19. H. Tournely, *Theologia Moralis* (Venetiis, 1756), Tom. III, Tract. De Decalogo, cap. 2. de Quinto Praec., Art. I, conc. 2, in Cronin, *The Moral Law*, 67. C. Roncaglia divided surgical procedures into categories separating those involving intense pain from those only involving moderate pain. He considered only intense pain to involve a moral impossibility to accept, and thus he admitted the necessity for a person to undergo moderate pain to conserve his life. C. Roncaglia, *Theologia Moralis* (Lucae, 1730), Vol. I, Tract. XI, Cap. I, Q. III.

20. John Gury, A. Ballerini, and D. Palmieri, *Compendium Theologiae Moralis* (ed. 14; Rome, 1907), I, nn. 389–91, in Cronin, *The Moral Law*, 78.

21. A. Ballerini, *Opus Theologicum Morale in Busenbaum Medullam, absolvit et edidit D. Palmieri* (Prati, 1899), II, 645, n. 868, n. b, in Gerald Kelly, SJ, "The Duty of Using Artificial Means of Preserving Life," *Theological Studies* 11.2 (June 1950): 205.

22. C. Capellmann, *Medicina Pastoralis*, 13th ed. (Aquisgrana, 1901).

23. II. Noldin and A. Schmitt, *Summa Theologiae Moralis*, 27th ed. (1941), vol. II, no. 328, cited in O'Donnell, *Medicine and Christian Morality*, 58.

24. O'Donnell, *Medicine and Christian Morality*, 58–59.

25. Kelly, "The Duty of Using Artificial Means of Preserving Life," 203.

26. See Joseph B. McAllister, *Ethics, with Special Application to the Medical and Nursing Professions*, 2nd ed. (Philadelphia: W. B. Saunders, 1955), 175. See also Cronin, *The Moral Law*, 91. A contradictory position can be found as far back as Francisco de Vitoria. Daniel Cronin wrote that Vitoria understood that "medicines and drugs—in fact artificial means in general—are intended by nature to supplement the natural means of conserving life. They are intended to help man to conserve his life when the use of merely natural means, such as food, sunshine, rest, etc., are not sufficient because of the individual's physical condition." In this way, according to Cronin's assessment of Vitoria, artificial means could be obligatory.

27. O'Donnell, *Medicine and Christian Morality*, 60.

28. Kelly, "The Duty of Using Artificial Means of Preserving Life," 213–14. John Connery questioned the use of the phrase "reasonable hope of success" used by Kelly. He said: "The question I would raise, tying this point to the previous one is this: Could one ever in the case of terminal illness, even though someone were not a grave burden, discontinue feeding him because there was not a 'reasonable hope of success' if he were fed normally? While most would consider this to be active euthanasia, it would seem possible to accept it within traditional Catholic thought, i.e., if natural means can sometimes be extraordinary, and extraordinary means are determined at times by usefulness, why not discontinue natural means if they are useless?" in Connery, "Prolonging Life," 222.

29. Kelly, "The Duty of Using Artificial Means of Preserving Life," 214. See also Atkinson, "Theological History of Catholic Teaching," 109.

30. Kelly, "The Duty of Using Artificial Means of Preserving Life," 214.

31. Cronin, *The Moral Law*, 94. He further stated: "God intends the development of science for the good of man. When science can provide a means of conserving man's life which can be a supplement to a natural means, then this artificial means would seem to be obligatory. It is true, however, that whereas natural means in general are ordinary means, artificial means of conserving life can quite often be extraordinary means and thus not obligatory. When artificial means are ordinary means, then they are obligatory."

32. Atkinson, "Theological History of Catholic Teaching," 108. See also James J. McCartney, OSA, "The Development of the Doctrine of Ordinary and Extraordinary Means of Preserving Life in Catholic Moral Theology Before the Karen Quinlan Case," *Linacre Quarterly* 47.3 (August 1980): 218. Rev. McCartney brought up two important points concerning Kelly's assessment of the ordinary and extraordinary means: "First, [Kelly] introduces the principle of totality into the discussion and maintains that perhaps we should consider the patient's total condition before we decide whether a given means is ordinary or extraordinary. Thus, for example, he sees the possibility of a diabetic with terminal cancer not taking insulin as perhaps an extraordinary means. He also emphasizes that we must consider the rights and duties of relatives and physicians when evaluating whether a given means of conserving life is ordinary or extraordinary."

33. Gerald Kelly, SJ, "The Duty to Preserve Life," *Theological Studies* 12.4 (December 1951): 550.

34. Daniel Cronin, *The Moral Law*, 127–28. See also Elizabeth McMillan, RSM, "The Catholic Moral Tradition on Providing Food and Fluids," *Linacre Quarterly* 54.4 (November 1987), 56–57.

35. Cronin, *The Moral Law*, 128. See also 102, where he explained the difficulty of establishing an absolute norm, particularly for the ordinary means. He remarked: "There are many factors in this notion of relativity. For example, the age of an individual . . . The person's physical and psychological condition . . . His financial status . . . " See also O'Donnell, *Medicine and Christian Morality*, 62–64.

36. Kelly, "The Duty to Preserve Life," 550–51. See also Kevin O'Rourke and Dennis Brodeur, *Medical Ethics: Common Ground for Understanding*, vol. 2 (St. Louis, MO: Catholic Health Association, 1989), 127–28. They comment that "the theologians developing the Catholic tradition in regard to prolonging life did not seek to remove decisions of conscience from ailing individuals. Thus they did not compile a list of 'objective means' that were too painful, expensive, difficult, or embarrassing for everyone. Neither did they seek to determine what would constitute 'a significant length of time' to prolong life. Rather, they determined some generic reasons that would justify the choice of a good that indirectly led to death and called upon people to make the required specific applications."

37. Cronin, *The Moral Law*, 102–12.

38. Ibid., 100.

39. See H. Jone and U. Adelman, *Moral Theology* (Westminster, MD: Newman Press, 1948), n. 210, in Cronin, *The Moral Law*, 87. They commented: "They exempt even wealthy people from the necessity of going to a far-distant place or health resort. Even the wealthy would not be obliged to summon the best known physicians."

40. Cronin, *The Moral Law*, 108. The writings of Tournely and Roncaglia apply here.

41. Ibid., at 99–112. See also Atkinson, "Theological History of Catholic Teaching," 110–11.

42. Cronin, *The Moral Law*, 112–26.

43. See Kelly, "The Duty of Using Artificial Means of Preserving Life," 206.

44. Cronin, *The Moral Law*, 112–26. See also Atkinson, "Theological History of Catholic Teaching," 111.

45. Pius XII, "The Prolongation of Life," 395–96. See also Russell E. Smith, "Ordinary versus Extraordinary Means," in *Ethical Principle in Catholic Health Care*, ed. Edward J. Furton (Boston, MA: The National Catholic Bioethics Center, 1999), 90. Smith states that "in these four sentences, the Holy Father has summarized and ratified the theological tradition regarding the distinction between ordinary and extraordinary means. He does not embrace the 'clinical' definition of ordinary means as entirely normative for ethical evaluation. Rather, the Pope understands the distinction to be determined by the relevant circumstances of the case in its clinical and personal dimensions."

46. See Kevin O'Rourke, OP, Philip Boyle, OP, and Larry King, "The Brophy Case: The Use of Artificial Hydration and Nutrition," *Linacre Quarterly* 54.2 (May 1987): 66–68; Kevin O'Rourke, OP, "Should Nutrition and Hydration Be Provided to Permanently Unconscious and Other Mentally Disabled Persons?" *Issues in Law and Medicine* 5.2 (Fall 1989): 181–96; Richard A. McCormick, "Moral Considerations Ill Considered," *America* 166.9 (March 14, 1992): 214; Richard A. McCormick, "To Save or Let Die: The Dilemma of Modern Medicine," *America* 131.1 (July 13, 1974): 8.

47. O'Rourke, "Should Nutrition and Hydration Be Provided," 188. Other theologians disagreed with the interpretation given to Pius XII's 1957 statement. Among those who disagreed is Orville Griese, "Pope Pius XII and 'Medical Treatments,'" *Linacre Quarterly* 54.4 (November 1987): 43–49.

48. Bryan Jennett, *The Vegetative State: Medical Facts, Ethical and Legal Dilemmas* (West Nyack, NY: Cambridge University Press, 2002), 105. Paul Ramsey proposed, particularly in the case of incompetents, a shift in terminology from "ordinary" and "extraordinary" to a medical indications norm. If a treatment was medically indicated in a certain situation, it was obligatory; if it was not medically indicated, then it would be non-obligatory or optional. See Paul Ramsey, *Ethics at the Edges of Life: Medical and Legal Intersections* (New Haven, CT: Yale University Press, 1978), 153–60. Robert Veatch made another proposal. His solution to the question of preserving life was to base treatment decisions on what was reasonable to the patient. See Robert Veatch, *Death, Dying, and the Biological Revolution: Our Last Quest for Responsibility* (New Haven, CT: Yale University Press, 1976), 77–115.

49. Congregation for the Doctrine of the Faith, *Declaration on Euthanasia* (May 5, 1980), *Origins* 10.10 (August 14, 1980): 156. See also Smith, "Ordinary versus Extraordinary Means," 89–90. As far back as Augustinus Lehmkuhl, SJ, the distinction between the theological understanding of the ordinary and extraordinary means and the medical interpretation of the same has been a part of the Catholic tradition. Fr. Lehmkuhl maintained that a person need not undergo a treatment involving pain, horror, or revulsion, even if that treatment was medically considered an ordinary means of conserving life. See Cronin, *The Moral Law*, 81; and Augustinus Lehmkuhl, *Theologica Moralis*, 10th ed. (Freiburg-im-Breisgau: Herder, 1902), 345.

50. O'Donnell, *Medicine and Christian Morality*, 65.

51. Both the Pontifical Academy of Sciences and the Pontifical Council for Pastoral Assistance considered the provision of AAHN an example of normal care. See Pontifical Academy

of Sciences, "The Artificial Prolongation of Life," *Origins* 15.25 (December 5, 1985): 415. The original document can be found in *Enchiridion Vaticanum*, IX (Bologna, Italy: Edizioni Dehoniane Bologna, 1987), 1727, n. 1768. See also Pontifical Council for Pastoral Assistance, *Charter for Health Care Workers* (Boston, MA: Daughters of St. Paul, 1995), n. 120.

52. Robert L. Barry, OP, gave the most detailed explanation for the argument that AAHN was an aspect of normal care. He argued that, in the circumstances in which tube feeding alone would maintain the life of a person in PVS, it was an aspect of basic nursing care, and not a medical treatment. See Robert Barry, OP, "Feeding the Comatose and the Common Good in the Catholic Tradition," *The Thomist* 53.1 (January 1989): 1–30. See also Robert L. Barry, OP, *The Sanctity of Human Life and Its Protection* (Lanham, MD: University Press of America, 2002), 151–52. Further, see Gilbert Meilaender, "On Removing Food and Water: Against the Stream," in *Bioethics: Basic Writings on the Key Ethical Questions that Surround the Major, Modern Biological Possibilities and Problems*, ed. Thomas A. Shannon, 3rd ed. (Mahwah, NJ: Paulist Press, 1987), 215–22.

53. Barry, *The Sanctity of Human Life and Its Protection* (Lanham, MD: University Press of America, 2002), 152.

54. Pennsylvania Bishops, "Nutrition and Hydration: Moral Considerations," *Origins* 21.34 (January 30, 1992): 548. See also U.S. Bishops' Pro-Life Committee, "Nutrition and Hydration: Moral and Pastoral Reflections," *Origins* 21.44 (April 9, 1992): 707. The Pro-Life Committee stated: "Even medical 'treatments' are morally obligatory when they are 'ordinary' means—that is, if they provide a reasonable hope of benefit and do not involve excessive burdens." See also U.S. Conference of Catholic Bishops, "Ethical and Religious Directives for Catholic Health Care Services, *Origins* 24.27 (December 15, 1994), 459, nn. 56–58.

55. Pennsylvania Bishops, "Nutrition and Hydration," 548. See also U.S. Bishops' Pro-Life Committee, "Nutrition and Hydration," 707–8. See also Mark Siegler, "Hydration and Nutrition: Medical, Legal, and Ethical Obligations," in *Scarce Medical Resources and Justice* (Braintree, MA: The Pope John XXIII Medical-Moral Research and Education Center, 1987), 134. He commented: "Should a relatively simple and ordinary medical and nursing intervention—specifically, the provision of fluid and nutritional support—be withheld by doctors and nurses from patients who are not terminally ill and who are not likely to die in a short time?"

56. U.S. Bishops' Pro-Life Committee, "Nutrition and Hydration," 708. They stated: "The difficulties families may face in this regard, and their need for improved financial and other assistance from the rest of society, should not be underestimated. While caring for a helpless loved one can provide many intangible benefits to family members and bring them closer together, the responsibilities of care can also strain even close and loving family relationships; complex medical decisions must be made under emotionally difficult circumstances not easily appreciated by those who have never faced such situations: 'Even here, however, we must try to think through carefully what we intend by withdrawing medically assisted nutrition and hydration. Are we deliberately trying to make sure that the patient dies in order to relieve caregivers of the financial and emotional burdens that will fall upon them if the patient survives? . . . Does my decision aim at relieving the patient of a particularly grave burden imposed by medically assisted nutrition and hydration? Or does it aim to avoid the total burden of caring for the patient? If so, does it achieve this aim by deliberately bringing about his or her death?'" See also William E. May et al., "Feeding and Hydrating the Permanently Unconscious and Other Vulnerable Persons," *Issues in Law*

and Medicine 3.3 (Winter 1987), 210. The authors commented: "The question remains whether providing food and water in this way to these patients is excessively burdensome because of its cost. At the outset we make two critical points. First, the cost of providing food and fluids by enteral tubes is not, in itself, excessive. Such feeding is generally no more costly than other forms of ordinary nursing care (such as cleaning or spoon-feeding a patient) or ordinary maintenance care (such as the maintenance of room temperature through heating or air conditioning). Second, one must also take into account the benefits that such care may provide both to the patient and to the caregivers." See also William E. May, *Catholic Bioethics and the Gift of Human Life* (Huntington, IN: Our Sunday Visitor Press, 2000), 268–69. He stated: "We granted that the total cost of caring for PVS patients (providing them with a heated room, nursing care, etc.) could be quite great, but that in our affluent society, which provides similar care for other persons in severely compromised positions (e.g., those who must be institutionalized because of chronic but nonfatal illnesses, etc.), it would be unfair and unjust to deprive the permanently unconscious of their fair share."

57. Pennsylvania Bishops, "Nutrition and Hydration," 549. See also U.S. Bishops' Pro-Life Committee, "Nutrition and Hydration," 708, and Germain Grisez, "Difficult Moral Questions: May a Husband End All Care of His Permanently Unconscious Wife?" *Linacre Quarterly* 63.2 (May 1996): 45.

58. Pontifical Council for Pastoral Assistance, *Charter for Health Care Workers*, n. 64.

59. Congregation for the Doctrine of the Faith, *Declaration on Euthanasia*, 156. The Congregation stated that "According to Christian teaching, however, suffering, especially suffering during the last moments of life, has a special place in God's saving plan; it is in fact a sharing in Christ's passion and a union with the redeeming sacrifice which he offered in obedience to the Father's will."

5

Must We Preserve Life?

Ronald Hamel

Michael Panicola

Is the removal of a feeding tube that supplies nutrients and fluids, especially in patients in a persistent vegetative state (PVS), simply a means of killing a vulnerable person—a form of euthanasia? Judging from some of the responses to the much-publicized Terri Schiavo case, it seems there are those who think so, including a fair number of Catholics. (Ms. Schiavo, a thirty-nine-year-old Florida resident, suffered severe brain damage after a collapse in 1990 and has been sustained since then by a feeding tube. Her husband has sought the removal of life-sustaining equipment. This is opposed by her parents and family, and the issue has been litigated for over five years.)

It is not always clear whether those who oppose removal of the feeding tube do so because they believe it is killing in this particular case or that it is killing in most or all such cases. In any event, the Terri Schiavo case has generated not only enormous controversy but also considerable confusion among Catholics and others regarding the moral justification for forgoing artificial nutrition and hydration.

The confusion, however, did not originate with the Terri Schiavo case. Reactions to other high-profile feeding-tube cases over the last twenty years or so have also contributed to the confusion. In general, this confusion has arisen because differing viewpoints have been expressed by church-related bodies discussing Catholic teaching on the duty to preserve life by providing nutrition and hydration (e.g., statements by the New Jersey and Texas bishops). More seriously, many of the statements that have been issued since the Vatican's *Declaration on Euthanasia* (1980) appear to revise and apply in a narrow way traditional Catholic teaching on the matter. In what follows, we offer a brief sketch of the tradition, then consider the two principal ways in which the tradition is being revised and, finally, reflect on the implications of these revisions.

Traditional Catholic Teaching

The Catholic tradition on the duty to preserve life has developed over the course of some five hundred years. Two Jesuit moralists, John J. Paris and the late Richard A. McCormick, presented an excellent summary of this tradition as it relates to the use of nutrition and hydration (*America*, May 2, 1987). We would like to highlight three important features of that summary for background purposes.

Duty to preserve life. The bedrock for the traditional teaching is found in the basic Christian understanding of life and death. As Christians we believe human life is a great good that has been given to us freely out of love by God, and through life we are able to enter more fully into communion with God by loving others. We therefore have a duty to protect and to preserve our lives. Yet this duty is not absolutely binding under all circumstances because we know our ultimate end lies in eternal life with God. Just what circumstances might relieve us of our duty to preserve life is a question that has been given considerable attention in the tradition.

It has been widely accepted among Catholic moralists since the sixteenth century that one need only employ "ordinary" means of preserving life but not means that are deemed "extraordinary" by which is meant measures that either fail to offer a proportionate hope of benefit or that impose an excessive burden. This distinction between ordinary and extraordinary means was first articulated explicitly by Dominican moralist Domingo Bañez (1528–1604) and it is still operative today, though now the terms proportionate and disproportionate are more often used.

The relative norm. There has been a shift away from the traditional terms because the meaning of *ordinary* and *extraordinary* began to be seriously misunderstood as medicine became more advanced and certain means of preserving life became more commonly used and readily available. As a consequence, the moral question regarding the effects of a particular therapeutic means upon a person in terms of benefits or burdens was reduced to a technical question about the means itself. If the means, without respect to the overall impact on the person, were an ordinary medical procedure or therapy, it was wrongly deemed ordinary in the moral sense of the term and hence obligatory. For the traditional moralists, however, no means of preserving life could be considered ordinary apart from an assessment of the benefits or burdens relative to the person's overall situation.

That this is true can be seen in the most comprehensive historical study of the topic, the 1958 doctoral dissertation of Daniel A. Cronin, who is now archbishop emeritus of Hartford, Connecticut. In discussing how one judges whether a means is ordinary and hence obligatory, Archbishop Cronin stated:

> the notion of proportionate hope of success and benefit is an essential part of the nature of ordinary means. Without this hope of benefit, a means is hardly an ordinary means and therefore is not obligatory. In determining the presence of this hope of success and benefit, one must consider not only the nature of the particular remedy or means involved, but also the relative condition of the person who is to use this means. Then, and then only, can the moral obligation of using such a means be properly determined.

This relative understanding of means is also seen in recent authoritative statements. In the *Declaration on Euthanasia,* for instance, we read: "It will be possible to make a correct judgment as to the means by studying the type of treatment to be used, its degree of complexity or risk, its cost and the possibilities of using it, and comparing these elements with the result that can be expected, taking into account the state of the sick person and his or her physical and moral resources." Likewise, Pope John Paul II stated in his encyclical letter *Evangelium Vitae* (1995): "Certainly there is a moral obligation to care for oneself and to allow oneself to be cared for, but this duty must take account of concrete circumstances. It needs to be determined whether the means of treatment available are objectively proportionate to the prospects for improvement."

Nutrition and hydration. Obviously the traditional Catholic moralists did not have to contend with questions about feeding tubes. But they did consider the moral obligation one has to preserve one's life with food and fluids. Given what was said above, it will not be surprising to learn that even such mundane means as food and fluids could be forgone if they failed to provide a proportionate hope of benefit or imposed excessive burdens. The Dominican moralist Francisco de Vitoria (1486–1546) made this clear when he argued that "if the depression of spirit is so low and there is present such consternation in the appetitive power that only with the greatest of effort and as though by means of a certain torture, can the sick man take food, right away that is reckoned a certain impossibility, and therefore he is excused, at least from mortal sin, especially where there is little hope of life or none at all."

De Vitoria's views were not unique among traditional moralists, nor were they subsequently rejected by contemporary ones. This is evident in the article "The Duty of Using Artificial Means of Preserving Life," published by the Jesuit moralist Gerald Kelly (1902–64) in *Theological Studies* in June 1950. In discussing whether oxygen and intravenous feeding must be used to preserve the life of a patient in a terminal coma, Kelly stated:

> I see no reason why even the most delicate professional standard should call for their use. In fact, it seems to me that, apart from very special circumstances, the artificial means not only need not but should not be used, once the coma is reasonably diagnosed as terminal. Their use creates expense and nervous strain without conferring any real benefit.

Revisions of the Teaching

By all accounts, the Catholic tradition on the duty to preserve life remained substantively the same from the early sixteenth century through the Holy See's *Declaration on Euthanasia* in 1980. But since then there has been a concerted effort by some to revise traditional Catholic teaching on the use of nutrition and hydration generally, and particularly in its application to patients in a persistent vegetative state. This has been done in two significant ways. The advocates of revision claim that nutrition and hydration are always obligatory, and they severely limit the meaning of the term benefit.

Nutrition and hydration always obligatory. Some of those attempting to revise the tradition define artificial nutrition and hydration as care, basic care or minimal measures for sustaining life and then assert that providing this care is always morally obligatory. For example, in its 1981 document, "Questions of Ethics Regarding the Fatally Ill and Dying," the Pontifical Council on Health Affairs stated: "there remains the strict obligation to apply *under all circumstances* those therapeutic measures which are called 'minimal': that is, those which are normally and customarily used for the maintenance of life (alimentation, blood transfusions, injections, etc.). To interrupt these *minimal measures* would, in practice, be equivalent to wishing to put an end to the patient's life" (emphasis added).

Similarly, in the "Report of the Pontifical Academy of Sciences on the Artificial Prolongation of Life" (1985), we find the statement: "If the patient is in a permanent, irreversible coma all *care* should be lavished on him, *including feeding*" (emphasis added). The New Jersey Catholic Conference, in its 1987 statement, "Providing Food and Fluids to Severely Brain Damaged Patients," also maintained that "nutrition and hydration, being *basic to human life*, are aspects of *normal care*, which are not excessively burdensome, that should *always be provided* to a patient" (emphasis added). Forgoing these means "ultimately results in starvation, dehydration, and death. It is direct. It is unnatural, as unnatural as denying one the air needed to breathe, or murder by asphyxiation."

This distinction between care and treatment seems to be a new development; the closest thing to it in the tradition is the distinction between natural and artificial means, which is morally irrelevant, as we will see. Certainly dying persons must always be cared for in ways that respect their inherent dignity. Traditionally, however, this has not meant that food and fluids must always be provided. The traditional moralists understood that even the most common or natural means of preserving life could be extraordinary and hence morally optional. Archbishop Cronin made this clear: "even the older moralists teach that such a purely ordinary and common means of conserving life as food admits of relative inconvenience and difficulty. Furthermore, they point out that this very common means, food, sometimes can offer no proportionate hope of success relative to a particular individual."

If this could be said of food and fluids, it would seem to apply all the more to various forms of artificial nutrition and hydration delivered through IV lines, nasogastric tubes, and gastrostomies. For the traditional moralists, the decisive moral consideration was not how basic a particular means was to life or how commonly or easily available it was. Rather, it was whether the means offered a proportionate hope of benefit without imposing excessive burdens relative to the person's overall situation.

We point out, as an aside here, that it seems logically inconsistent to classify nutrition and hydration as basic care that is always obligatory even if artificially supplied while not doing the same for oxygen supplied by mechanical ventilation or other basic elements of care necessary for life. Why does nutrition and hydration merit such a classification? As we see it, the case for doing so has not only not been adequately made; it has not been argued at all.

Meaning of "benefit" severely restricted. Some of those attempting to revise the tradition also restrict the notion of benefit simply to the preservation of physical life itself. For example, in "Nutrition and Hydration: Moral and Pastoral Reflections," the U.S. Bishops' Pro-Life Committee commented in 1992 that "[nutrition and hydration] must not be withdrawn in order to cause death, but they may be withdrawn if they offer no reasonable hope of *sustaining life* or pose excessive risks or burdens" (emphasis added).

In a qualitatively major shift, the Pro-Life Committee replaced the traditional language of proportionate hope of benefit relative to the person with "reasonable hope of sustaining life." The Florida Catholic Conference similarly restricted the notion of benefit in much the same way, albeit in negative terms, in its statement regarding Terri Schiavo: "Bishop Lynch's statement clarifies the teaching of the Church that nourishment or hydration may be withheld or withdrawn where that treatment itself is causing harm to the patient or *is useless because the patient's death is imminent*" (emphasis added). The assumption here appears to be that nutrition and hydration naturally or artificially supplied are always beneficial, except when they fail to sustain life because death is inevitable regardless of what is done.

This limited physical understanding of benefit is not the way traditional moralists understood it. The mere fact that a means was capable of sustaining life did not necessarily mean it was beneficial to the person. De Vitoria argued this point when he stated "that one is not held to lengthen his life, because he is not held to use always the most delicate foods, that is, hens and chickens, even though he has the ability and the doctors say that if he eats in such a manner, *he will live 20 years more*; and even if he knew this for certain, he would not be obliged" (emphasis added).

Admittedly, the meaning of *benefit* is hard to define because of the relative factors involved. One thing is certain, however: The traditional moralists did not restrict benefit merely to sustaining life but included broader, more holistic considerations. Improvements in one's condition, relief of pain, maximization of comfort, restoration of health, among others—all were considered beneficial. Yet, as we read the tradition, these physical effects were beneficial insofar as they enabled one to pursue human goods bound up with physical life and spiritual goods that transcend it, at least at a minimal level, without imposing excessive burdens. This explains why De Vitoria said that even a means that could sustain life for another twenty years would not be morally obligatory. For De Vitoria and other traditional moralists, the mere preservation of physical life and vital physiological functions was not sufficient in itself to oblige someone to use a certain means, including food and fluids.

From our quick review of the Catholic tradition on the duty to preserve life and some recent church statements on nutrition and hydration, we can see that the traditional teaching is being revised. In essence, two standards for making decisions about nutrition and hydration have emerged and now exist side by side. One is a more holistic standard based on the traditional teaching, in which benefits and burdens are understood broadly relative to the person, and any means of preserving life is subject to a benefit–burden analysis. The other is a more restrictive standard based on recent revisions of the traditional teaching in which benefits and burdens are understood narrowly, apart from relative factors, and nutrition and hydration are given a special moral classification.

Proof of this can be seen in the fourth edition of *Ethical and Religious Directives for Catholic Health Care Services*, published in 2001 by the U.S. Conference of Catholic Bishops to provide authoritative ethical guidance to Catholic health care providers. The introduction to part 6, for instance, states the more restrictive standard: "These statements agree that hydration and nutrition are not morally obligatory either when they *bring no comfort* to a person who is *imminently dying* or when they *cannot be assimilated* by the person's body" (emphasis added).

In all the opinions we have considered from the traditional moralists and in all of our studies of the tradition, nowhere do we see the exceptional circumstances under which one may morally forgo a means of preserving life reduced to imminent death or futility simply because it will not work. For the traditional moralists, these were the easy cases. What they strained over and worked out was a practical moral standard for the gray-area cases, of which we see shades in the latter part of *ERD* Directive 58: "There should be a presumption in favor of providing nutrition and hydration to all patients, including patients who require medically assisted nutrition and hydration, as long as this is *of sufficient benefit to outweigh the burdens involved to the patient*" (emphasis added). Here benefits and burdens are not explicitly defined in a narrow way. When this directive is read against the backdrop of Directives 56 and 57 on the definitions of ordinary and extraordinary means, the *ERD* returns to the more traditional understanding.

Two Standards

The confusion among Catholics about the church's teaching on forgoing artificial nutrition and hydration, as evidenced by the Terri Schiavo case and others like it, is due largely to the fact that we now have two standards for making decisions. What are we to make of this? Could it be that we are experiencing a development of church teaching toward the more restrictive standard? This might be.

In 1998, Pope John Paul II lent credence to the view that nutrition and hydration are ordinary or proportionate means, and hence morally obligatory, when he stated during an *ad limina* visit in Rome by U.S. bishops from California, Hawaii, and Nevada that "a great teaching effort is needed to clarify the substantive moral difference between discontinuing medical procedures that may be burdensome, dangerous, or disproportionate to the expected outcome and taking away the *ordinary means* of preserving life, such as *feeding, hydration and normal medical care*" (emphasis added).

The pope seemed to go further in an audience in March 2004, speaking to participants in an international conference on nutrition and hydration and the vegetative state that was sponsored by the World Federation of Catholic Medical Associations and the Pontifical Academy for Life. On that occasion the pope stated that "sick people in a vegetative state, waiting to recover or for a natural end, have the right to basic health care (nutrition, hydration, hygiene, warmth, etc)."

He went on to "underline how the administration of water and food, even when provided by artificial means, always represents a *natural means* of preserving life, not a *medical act*. Its use, furthermore, should be considered, in principle, *ordinary and proportionate*, and as such morally obligatory, insofar as and until it is seen to have attained its proper finality, which in the present case consists in providing nourishment to the patient and alleviation of his suffering" (emphasis in original).

It is not entirely clear at this time what the implications of these papal statements are for Catholic patients, families, caregivers and health care organizations. Some believe that by his latest statement, the pope has made nutrition and hydration morally obligatory for all patients under all circumstances and has thus altered a tradition of more than five hundred years. But an alternative reading is also possible. Although the pope definitely narrows traditional teaching by claiming that nutrition and hydration are ordinary, apart from relative factors, he does not radically and completely depart from traditional understandings or his own previous teachings by making their use an absolute requirement with no exceptions. If the pope's statement is read in light of the tradition, what he might be saying is that *in principle* nutrition and hydration are ordinary means of preserving life and hence morally obligatory for all patients. This appears to be just a continuation of what we have seen already in the U.S. bishops' Pro-Life Committee document of 1992 and in Directive 58, where we hear of a presumption in favor of providing nutrition and hydration.

Were the pope going beyond this presumption and arguing instead for an absolute requirement, he would not likely have uttered the phrase "*insofar as* and until it is seen to have attained its proper finality" (emphasis added). Here the pope may be indicating that nutrition and hydration are not always obligatory but only to the extent that they serve their ultimate purpose. Furthermore, and most important, the pope goes on to specify just what this proper finality is— but *only* for patients in a PVS. He does this by saying, "which in *the present case* consists in providing nourishment to the patient and alleviation of suffering" (emphasis added). The "present case" refers to those in a PVS, which was the focus of the conference and of the pope's statement read at the conclusion of the conference. So we may well be left with a presumption in favor of providing nutrition and hydration to all patients. But nutrition and hydration can be withheld or withdrawn when they do not attain their proper finality, which for patients in general can be decided on traditional grounds (i.e., holistic benefit–burden analysis) and for patients in a PVS on the more limited grounds set by the pope (i.e., nourishment *and* alleviation of suffering).

Whatever the pope intended to say about the particulars of caring for PVS patients, his general purpose for making the statement seems clear. He has spoken frequently about a "culture of death" that pervades modern society. In that context, he seems especially worried that forgoing nutrition and hydration from vulnerable patients (e.g., those in a PVS) could easily degenerate into euthanasia. The documents to which we have referred and others as well echo this concern. The New Jersey Catholic Conference document, for example, states: "Today food and nutrition is withdrawn from someone in a persistent comatose state; tomorrow such care is withdrawn from someone suffering from Alzheimer's disease."

The concern is legitimate, especially with regard to those who are unable to speak for themselves. Undoubtedly, forgoing life-sustaining treatment, including artificial nutrition and hydration, can be abused. It can take the form of euthanasia. The possibility that this will happen is perhaps greater than ever today, with physician-assisted suicide (PAS) gaining wider support and our collective appreciation for life eroding. But we must all carefully consider whether a narrow revision and application of the tradition is the most effective response to this threat. Instead of limiting abuse, such a narrowing could have the opposite effect. It could, in fact, propel requests for PAS and euthanasia. Let us not forget that the reasons for requesting PAS center on fear of dying in pain, fear of being a burden to others, or fear of having life unreasonably prolonged.

Furthermore, such a revision has no hope of being effective if it does not resonate with the best of human experience and if it is not persuasive. To date, the case for restricting the forgoing of artificial nutrition and hydration has not been adequately made. Nor have the statements proposing such a restriction addressed modern medical evidence showing that artificial nutrition and hydration are not always beneficial and can impose serious burdens on the patient. A more restrictive standard crafted in light of exceptional cases does not seem indicated, given the medical evidence to the contrary. Moreover, such a standard is not supported from a biological standpoint since most dying persons naturally stop eating and drinking.

Perhaps a more constructive approach to securing the dignity of the dying and preventing abuses is not to react to the negative possibilities. A better approach might be to seek to transform our contemporary culture by honoring the traditional teaching and developing quality palliative care programs that can address the holistic needs of seriously ill and dying persons as well as the concerns of their families. Witnessing to the dignity of those who are approaching the mystery of death is likely to have a far greater transformative effect on attitudes toward the dying and the vulnerable than restricting or narrowing our centuries-long tradition in ways that could well impose additional burdens on these patients and their families. It may be that neither this consideration nor any other would have helped resolve the Terri Schiavo case, given the great divide between her loved ones. However, in the majority of cases involving decisions to forgo nutrition and hydration or any other means of preserving life, the traditional teaching and a comprehensive palliative care strategy will be effective Christian witness to our basic understanding of life and death.

PART THREE

Ecclesiastical and Pastoral Perspectives

Over the past fifty years, the magisterium and various episcopal bodies have addressed the Catholic moral tradition on the duty to preserve life and forgoing life-sustaining treatment. This section offers a sampling of these statements.

Two of the most important statements are Pope Pius XII's 1957 address to anesthesiologists and the Congregation for the Doctrine of the Faith's 1980 *Declaration on Euthanasia*. Both documents reiterate familiar themes from the theological tradition although the *Declaration on Euthanasia* breaks some new ground by introducing the terms "proportionate" and "disproportionate" means as alternatives to "ordinary" and "extraordinary" means. Both of these documents solidified longstanding ethical reflection and practice with regard to forgoing or withdrawing life-sustaining treatment.

Subsequent to the publication of the *Declaration on Euthanasia*, most likely in direct and indirect response to a number of high-visibility cases involving patients in PVS, several Vatican advisory bodies and several state Catholic conferences issued statements applying the traditional teaching about forgoing or withdrawing life-sustaining treatment to artificial nutrition and hydration, particularly regarding patients in PVS. In addition to the report of the Pontifical Academy of Sciences' study group included in this section, there were also statements by the Pontifical Council *Cor Unum* ("Questions of Ethics Regarding the Fatally Ill and Dying," 1981) and the Pontifical Council for Pastoral Assistance to Health Care Workers (*Charter for Health Care Workers*, 1995). The statements by the Texas Catholic Bishops and Texas Conference of Catholic Health Facilities as well as the USCCB Committee for Pro-Life Activities, both included in this section, are examples of how bishops in the United States weighed in on the matter. Other state bishops' conferences also issued statements—New Jersey (1987), Oregon and Washington (1991), and Pennsylvania (1992).

These pastoral statements do not reflect a univocal perspective in their understanding or application of traditional teaching. Instead, they reveal some of the elements of different approaches to assessing the moral justifiability of forgoing or withdrawing artificial nutrition and hydration that currently exist. The differences among them center on such critical issues as how one views human life and its relation to eternal life, how one determines whether an intervention is ordinary or extraordinary, how benefit and burden are understood, what is deemed to be the cause of death, and the matter of intention in forgoing or withdrawing artificial nutrition and hydration. An underlying and broader question is how these various understandings compare with the theological tradition and the teaching of the magisterium as reflected in the statement of Pius XII and the *Declaration on Euthanasia.*

The different approaches are evident in the last selection in this section—a portion of part 5 of *The Ethical and Religious Directives for Catholic Health Care Services*—a document issued by the United States Conference of Catholic Bishops that guides the practice of Catholic health care organizations. The discussion of artificial nutrition and hydration in the introduction to part 5 (and, to some degree, Directive 58) differs from the principles enunciated in Directive 56 (proportionate means) and Directive 57 (disproportionate means). In the introduction and in Directive 58, there seems to be an attempt to accommodate differing views and to give expression to an alternative view that began to emerge in 1981.

What is to be made of these differing approaches to forgoing or withdrawing artificial nutrition and hydration, especially in patients in PVS? Does the more recent approach represent a development in the Catholic moral tradition, or a departure from that tradition? This question has yet to be answered; it is part of the ongoing theological debate over this issue.

6

The Prolongation of Life

Pope Pius XII

Dr. Bruno Haid, chief of the anesthesia section at the surgery clinic of the University of Innsbruck, has submitted to Us three questions on medical morals treating the subject known as "resuscitation" [*la réanimation*].

We are pleased, gentlemen, to grant this request, which shows your great awareness of professional duties, and your will to solve in the light of the principles of the Gospel the delicate problems that confront you.

Problems of Anesthesiology

According to Dr. Haid's statement, modern anesthesiology deals not only with problems of analgesia and anesthesia properly so-called, but also with those of "resuscitation." This is the name given in medicine, and especially in anesthesiology, to the technique which makes possible the remedying of certain occurrences which seriously threaten human life, especially asphyxia, which formerly, when modern anesthetizing equipment was not yet available, would stop the heartbeat and bring about death in a few minutes. The task of the anesthesiologist has therefore extended to acute respiratory difficulties, provoked by strangulation or by open wounds of the chest. The anesthesiologist intervenes to prevent asphyxia resulting from the internal obstruction of breathing passages by the contents of the stomach or by drowning, to remedy total or partial respiratory paralysis in cases of serious tetanus, of poliomyelitis, of poisoning by gas, sedatives, or alcoholic intoxication, or even in cases of paralysis of the central respiratory apparatus caused by serious trauma of the brain.

The Practice of "Resuscitation"

In the practice of resuscitation and in the treatment of persons who have suffered head wounds, and sometimes in the case of persons who have undergone brain surgery or of those who have suffered trauma of the brain through anoxia and remain in a state of deep unconsciousness, there arise a number of questions that concern medical morality and involve the principles of the philosophy of nature even more than those of analgesia.

It happens at times—as in the aforementioned cases of accidents and illnesses, the treatment of which offers reasonable hope of success—that the anesthesiologist can improve the general condition of patients who suffer from a serious lesion of the brain and whose situation at first might seem desperate. He restores breathing either through manual intervention or with the help of special instruments, clears the breathing passages, and provides for the artificial feeding of the patient.

Thanks to this treatment, and especially through the administration of oxygen by means of artificial respiration, a failing blood circulation picks up again and the appearance of the patient improves, sometimes very quickly, to such an extent that the anesthesiologist himself, or any other doctor who, trusting his experience, would have given up all hope, maintains a slight hope that spontaneous breathing will be restored. The family usually considers this improvement an astonishing result and is grateful to the doctor.

If the lesion of the brain is so serious that the patient will very probably, and even most certainly, not survive, the anesthesiologist is then led to ask himself the distressing question as to the value and meaning of the resuscitation processes. As an immediate measure he will apply artificial respiration by intubation and by aspiration of the respiratory tract; he is then in a safer position and has more time to decide what further must be done. But he can find himself in a delicate position, if the family considers that the efforts he has taken are improper and opposes them. In most cases this situation arises, not at the beginning of resuscitation attempts, but when the patient's condition, after a slight improvement at first, remains stationary and it becomes clear that only automatic artificial respiration is keeping him alive. The question then arises if one must, or if one can, continue the resuscitation process despite the fact that the soul may already have left the body.

The solution to this problem, already difficult in itself, becomes even more difficult when the family—themselves Catholic perhaps—insist that the doctor in charge, especially the anesthesiologist, remove the artificial respiration apparatus in order to allow the patient, who is already virtually dead, to pass away in peace.

A Fundamental Problem

Out of this situation there arises a question that is fundamental, from the point of view of religion and the philosophy of nature. When, according to Christian faith, has death occurred in patients on whom modern methods of resuscitation have been used? Is Extreme Unction valid, at least as long as one can perceive heartbeats, even if the vital functions properly so-called have already disappeared, and if life depends only on the functioning of the artificial-respiration apparatus?

Three Questions

The problems that arise in the modern practice of resuscitation can therefore be formulated in three questions:

First, does one have the right, or is one even under the obligation, to use modern artificial-respiration equipment in all cases, even those which, in the doctor's judgment, are completely hopeless?

Second, does one have the right, or is one under obligation, to remove the artificial-respiration apparatus when, after several days, the state of deep unconsciousness does not improve if, when it is removed, blood circulation will stop within a few minutes? What must be done in this case if the family of the patient, who has already received the last sacraments, urges the doctor to remove the apparatus? Is Extreme Unction still valid at this time?

Third, must a patient plunged into unconsciousness through central paralysis, but whose life—that is to say, blood circulation—is maintained through artificial respiration, and in whom there is no improvement after several days, be considered "*de facto*" or even "*de jure*" dead? Must one not wait for blood circulation to stop, in spite of the artificial respiration, before considering him dead?

Basic Principles

We shall willingly answer these three questions. But before examining them, we would like to set forth the principles that will allow formulation of the answer.

Natural reason and Christian morals say that man (and whoever is entrusted with the task of taking care of his fellowman) has the right and the duty in case of serious illness to take the necessary treatment for the preservation of life and health. This duty that one has toward himself, toward God, toward the human community, and in most cases toward certain determined persons, derives from well ordered charity, from submission to the Creator, from social justice and even from strict justice, as well as from devotion toward one's family.

But normally one is held to use only ordinary means—according to circumstances of persons, places, times, and culture—that is to say, means that do not involve any grave burden for oneself or another. A more strict obligation would be too burdensome for most men and would render the attainment of the higher, more important good too difficult. Life, health, all temporal activities are in fact subordinated to spiritual ends. On the other hand, one is not forbidden to take more than the strictly necessary steps to preserve life and health, as long as he does not fail in some more serious duty.

Administration of the Sacraments

Where the administration of sacraments to an unconscious man is concerned, the answer is drawn from the doctrine and practice of the Church which, for its part, follows the Lord's will as its rule of action. Sacraments are meant, by virtue of divine institution, for men of this world who are in the course of their earthly life, and, except for baptism itself, presuppose prior baptism of the recipient. He who is not a man, who is not yet a man, or is no longer a man, cannot receive the sacraments. Furthermore, if someone expresses his refusal, the sacraments cannot be administered to him against his will. God compels no one to accept sacramental grace.

When it is not known whether a person fulfills the necessary conditions for valid reception of the sacraments, an effort must be made to solve the doubt. If this effort fails, the sacrament will be conferred under at least a tacit condition (with the phrase "*Si capax est*," "If you are capable,"—which is the broadest condition). Sacraments are instituted by Christ for men in order to save their souls.

Therefore, in cases of extreme necessity, the Church tries extreme solutions in order to give man sacramental grace and assistance.

The Fact of Death

The question of the fact of death and that of verifying the fact itself (*"de facto"*) or its legal authenticity (*"de jure"*) have, because of their consequences, even in the field of morals and of religion, an even greater importance. What we have just said about the presupposed essential elements for the valid reception of a sacrament has shown this. But the importance of the question extends also to effects in matters of inheritance, marriage and matrimonial processes, benefices (vacancy of a benefice), and to many other questions of private and social life.

It remains for the doctor, and especially the anesthesiologist, to give a clear and precise definition of "death" and the "moment of death" of a patient who passes away in a state of unconsciousness. Here one can accept the usual concept of complete and final separation of the soul from the body; but in practice one must take into account the lack of precision of the terms "body" and "separation." One can put aside the possibility of a person being buried alive, for removal of the artificial respiration apparatus must necessarily bring about stoppage of blood circulation and therefore death within a few minutes.

In case of insoluble doubt, one can resort to presumptions of law and of fact. In general, it will be necessary to presume that life remains, because there is involved here a fundamental right received from the Creator, and it is necessary to prove with certainty that it has been lost.

We shall now pass to the solution of the particular questions.

A Doctor's Rights and Duties

I. Does the anesthesiologist have the right, or is he bound, in all cases of deep unconsciousness, even in those that are considered to be completely hopeless in the opinion of the competent doctor, to use modern artificial respiration apparatus, even against the will of the family?

In ordinary cases one will grant that the anesthesiologist has the right to act in this manner, but he is not bound to do so, unless this becomes the only way of fulfilling another certain moral duty.

The rights and duties of the doctor are correlative to those of the patient. The doctor, in fact, has no separate or independent right where the patient is concerned. In general he can take action only if the patient explicitly or implicitly, directly or indirectly, gives him permission. The technique of resuscitation which concerns us here does not contain anything immoral in itself. Therefore the patient, if he were capable of making a personal decision, could lawfully use it and, consequently, give the doctor permission to use it. On the other hand, since these forms of treatment go beyond the ordinary means to which one is bound, it cannot be held that there is an obligation to use them nor, consequently, that one is bound to give the doctor permission to use them.

The rights and duties of the family depend in general upon the presumed will of the unconscious patient if he is of age and "*sui juris.*" Where the proper and independent duty of the family is concerned, they are usually bound only to the use of ordinary means.

Consequently, if it appears that the attempt at resuscitation constitutes in reality such a burden for the family that one cannot in all conscience impose it upon them, they can lawfully insist that the doctor should discontinue these attempts, and the doctor can lawfully comply. There is not involved here a case of direct disposal of the life of the patient, nor of euthanasia in any way: this would never be licit. Even when it causes the arrest of circulation, the interruption of attempts at resuscitation is never more than an indirect cause of the cessation of life, and one must apply in this case the principle of double effect and of "*voluntarium in causa.*"

Extreme Unction

2. We have, therefore, already answered the second question in essence: "Can the doctor remove the artificial respiration apparatus before the blood circulation has come to a complete stop? Can he do this, at least, when the patient has already received Extreme Unction? Is this Extreme Unction valid when it is administered at the moment when circulation ceases, or even after?"

We must give an affirmative answer to the first part of this question, as we have already explained. If Extreme Unction has not yet been administered, one must seek to prolong respiration until this has been done. But as far as concerns the validity of Extreme Unction at the moment when blood circulation stops completely or even after this moment, it is impossible to answer "yes" or "no."

If, as in the opinion of doctors, this complete cessation of circulation means a sure separation of the soul from the body, even if particular organs go on functioning, Extreme Unction would certainly not be valid, for the recipient would certainly not be a man anymore. And this is an indispensable condition for the reception of the sacraments.

If, on the other hand, doctors are of the opinion that the separation of the soul from the body is doubtful, and that this doubt cannot be solved, the validity of Extreme Unction is also doubtful. But, applying her usual rules: "The sacraments are for men" and "In case of extreme necessity one tries extreme measures," the Church allows the sacrament to be administered conditionally in respect to the sacramental sign.

When Is One "Dead"?

3. "When the blood circulation and the life of a patient who is deeply unconscious because of a central paralysis are maintained only through artificial respiration, and no improvement is noted after a few days, at what time does the Catholic Church consider the patient 'dead,' or when must he be declared dead according to natural law (questions '*de facto*' and '*dejure*')?"

(Has death already occurred after grave trauma of the brain, which has provoked deep unconsciousness and central breathing paralysis, the fatal consequences of which have nevertheless been retarded by artificial respiration? Or does it occur, according to the present opinion of doctors, only when there is complete arrest of circulation despite prolonged artificial respiration?)

Where the verification of the fact in particular cases is concerned, the answer cannot be deduced from any religious and moral principle and, under this aspect, does not fall within the competence of the Church. Until an answer can be given, the question must remain open. But considerations of a general nature allow us to believe that human life continues for as long as its vital functions—distinguished from the simple life of organs—manifest themselves spontaneously or even with the help of artificial processes. A great number of these cases are the object of insoluble doubt, and must be dealt with according to the presumptions of law and of fact of which we have spoken.

May these explanations guide you and enlighten you when you must solve delicate questions arising in the practice of your profession. As a token of divine favors which we call upon you and all those who are dear to you, we heartily grant you our Apostolic Blessing.

7

Declaration on Euthanasia

Sacred Congregation for the Doctrine of the Faith

Introduction

The rights and values pertaining to the human person occupy an important place among the questions discussed today. In this regard, the Second Vatican Ecumenical Council solemnly reaffirmed the lofty dignity of the human person, and in a special way his or her right to life. The Council therefore condemned crimes against life "such as any type of murder, genocide, abortion, euthanasia, or willful suicide" (Pastoral Constitution *Gaudium et Spes*, n. 27).

More recently, the Sacred Congregation for the Doctrine of the Faith has reminded all the faithful of Catholic teaching on procured abortion.[1] The Congregation now considers it opportune to set forth the Church's teaching on euthanasia.

It is indeed true that, in this sphere of teaching, the recent popes have explained the principles, and these retain their full force;[2] but the progress of medical science in recent years has brought to the fore new aspects of the question of euthanasia, and these aspects call for further elucidation on the ethical level.

In modern society, in which even the fundamental values of human life are often called into question, cultural change exercises an influence upon the way of looking at suffering and death; moreover, medicine has increased its capacity to cure and to prolong life in particular circumstances, which sometime give rise to moral problems. Thus people living in this situation experience no little anxiety about the meaning of advanced old age and death. They also begin to wonder whether they have the right to obtain for themselves or their fellowmen an "easy death," which would shorten suffering and which seems to them more in harmony with human dignity.

A number of Episcopal Conferences have raised questions on this subject with the Sacred Congregation for the Doctrine of the Faith. The Congregation, having sought the opinion of experts on the various aspects of euthanasia, now wishes to respond to the Bishops' questions with the present Declaration, in order to help them to give correct teaching to the faithful entrusted to their care, and to offer them elements for reflection that they can present to the civil authorities with regard to this very serious matter.

The considerations set forth in the present document concern in the first place all those who place their faith and hope in Christ, who, through His life, death, and resurrection, has given a new meaning to existence and especially to the death of the Christian, as St. Paul says: "If we live, we live to the Lord, and if we die, we die to the Lord" (Rom. 14:8; cf. Phil. 1:20).

As for those who profess other religions, many will agree with us that faith in God the Creator, Provider and Lord of life—if they share this belief—confers a lofty dignity upon every human person and guarantees respect for him or her.

It is hoped that this Declaration will meet with the approval of many people of good will, who, philosophical or ideological differences notwithstanding, have nevertheless a lively awareness of the rights of the human person. These rights have often, in fact, been proclaimed in recent years through declarations issued by International Congresses;[3] and since it is a question here of fundamental rights inherent in every human person, it is obviously wrong to have recourse to arguments from political pluralism or religious freedom in order to deny the universal value of those rights.

I. The Value of Human Life

Human life is the basis of all goods, and is the necessary source and condition of every human activity and of all society. Most people regard life as something sacred and hold that no one may dispose of it at will, but believers see in life something greater, namely, a gift of God's love, which they are called upon to preserve and make fruitful. And it is this latter consideration that gives rise to the following consequences:

1. No one can make an attempt on the life of an innocent person without opposing God's love for that person, without violating a fundamental right, and therefore without committing a crime of the utmost gravity.[4]
2. Everyone has the duty to lead his or her life in accordance with God's plan. That life is entrusted to the individual as a good that must bear fruit already here on earth but that finds its full perfection only in eternal life.
3. Intentionally causing one's own death, or suicide, is therefore equally as wrong as murder; such an action on the part of a person is to be considered as a rejection of God's sovereignty and loving plan. Furthermore, suicide is also often a refusal of love for self, the denial of a natural instinct to live, a flight from the duties of justice and charity owed to one's neighbor, to various communities or to the whole of society—although, as is generally recognized, at times there are psychological factors present that can diminish responsibility or even completely remove it.

However, one must clearly distinguish suicide from that sacrifice of one's life whereby for a higher cause, such as God's glory, the salvation of souls or the service of one's brethren, a person offers his or her own life or puts it in danger (cf. Jn. 15:14).

II. Euthanasia

In order that the question of euthanasia can be properly dealt with, it is first necessary to define the words used.

Etymologically speaking, in ancient times euthanasia meant an easy death without severe suffering. Today one no longer thinks of this original meaning of the word but rather of some intervention of medicine whereby the sufferings of sickness or of the final agony are reduced, sometimes also with the danger of suppressing life prematurely. Ultimately, the word euthanasia is used in a more particular sense to mean "mercy killing," for the purpose of putting an end to extreme suffering, or saving abnormal babies, the mentally ill or the incurably sick from the prolongation, perhaps for many years of a miserable life, which could impose too heavy a burden on their families or on society.

It is, therefore, necessary to state clearly in what sense the word is used in the present document.

By euthanasia is understood an action or an omission which of itself or by intention causes death in order that all suffering may in this way be eliminated.

Euthanasia's terms of reference, therefore, are to be found in the intention of the will and in the methods used.

It is necessary to state firmly once more that nothing and no one can in any way permit the killing of an innocent human being, whether a fetus or an embryo, an infant or an adult, an old person, or one suffering from an incurable disease, or a person who is dying. Furthermore, no one is permitted to ask for this act of killing, either for himself or herself or for another person entrusted to his or her care, nor can he or she consent to it, either explicitly or implicitly. Nor can any authority legitimately recommend or permit such an action. For it is a question of the violation of the divine law, an offense against the dignity of the human person, a crime against life, and an attack on humanity.

It may happen that, by reason of prolonged and barely tolerable pain, for deeply personal or other reasons, people may be led to believe that they can legitimately ask for death or obtain it for others. Although in these cases the guilt of the individual may be reduced or completely absent, nevertheless the error of judgment into which the conscience falls, perhaps in good faith, does not change the nature of this act of killing, which will always be in itself something to be rejected.

The pleas of gravely ill people who sometimes ask for death are not to be understood as implying a true desire for euthanasia; in fact, it is almost always a case of an anguished plea for help and love. What a sick person needs, besides medical care, is love, the human and supernatural warmth with which the sick person can and ought to be surrounded by all those close to him or her, parents and children, doctors and nurses.

III. The Meaning of Suffering for Christians and the Use of Painkillers

Death does not always come in dramatic circumstances after barely tolerable sufferings. Nor do we have to think only of extreme cases. Numerous testimonies which confirm one another lead one to the conclusion that nature itself has made provision to render more bearable at the moment of death separations that would be terribly painful to a person in full health. Hence it is that a prolonged illness, advanced old age, or a state of loneliness or neglect can bring about psychological conditions that facilitate the acceptance of death.

Nevertheless the fact remains that death, often preceded or accompanied by severe and prolonged suffering, is something which naturally causes people anguish.

Physical suffering is certainly an unavoidable element of the human condition; on the biological level, it constitutes a warning of which no one denies the usefulness; but, since it affects the human psychological makeup, it often exceeds its own biological usefulness and so can become so severe as to cause the desire to remove it at any cost.

According to Christian teaching, however, suffering, especially suffering during the last moments of life, has a special place in God's saving plan; it is in fact a sharing in Christ's passion and a union with the redeeming sacrifice which He offered in obedience to the Father's will. Therefore, one must not be surprised if some Christians prefer to moderate their use of painkillers, in order to accept voluntarily at least a part of their sufferings and thus associate themselves in a conscious way with the sufferings of Christ crucified (cf. Mt. 27:34).

Nevertheless it would be imprudent to impose a heroic way of acting as a general rule. On the contrary, human and Christian prudence suggest for the majority of sick people the use of medicines capable of alleviating or suppressing pain, even though these may cause as a secondary effect semiconsciousness and reduced lucidity. As for those who are not in a state to express themselves, one can reasonably presume that they wish to take these painkillers, and have them administered according to the doctor's advice.

But the intensive use of painkillers is not without difficulties because the phenomenon of habituation generally makes it necessary to increase their dosage in order to maintain their efficacy. At this point it is fitting to recall a declaration by Pius XII, which retains its full force; in answer to a group of doctors who had put the question: "Is the suppression of pain and consciousness by the use of narcotics . . . permitted by religion and morality to the doctor and the patient (even at the approach of death and if one foresees that the use of narcotics will shorten life)?"

The Pope said: "If no other means exist, and if, in the given circumstances, this does not prevent the carrying out of other religious and moral duties: Yes."[5] In this case, of course, death is in no way intended or sought, even if the risk of it is reasonably taken; the intention is simply to relieve pain effectively, using for this purpose painkillers available to medicine.

However, painkillers that cause unconsciousness need special consideration. For a person not only has to be able to satisfy his or her moral duties and family obligations; he or she also has to prepare himself or herself with full consciousness for meeting Christ. Thus Pius XII warns: "It is not right to deprive the dying person of consciousness without a serious reason."[6]

IV. Due Proportion in the Use of Remedies

Today it is very important to protect, at the moment of death, both the dignity of the human person and the Christian concept of life, against a technological attitude that threatens to become an abuse. Thus some people speak of a "right to die," which is an expression that does not mean the right to procure death either by one's own hand or by means of someone else, as one pleases, but rather the right to die peacefully with human and Christian dignity. From this point of view, the use of therapeutic means can sometimes pose problems.

In numerous cases, the complexity of the situation can be such as to cause doubts about the way ethical principles should be applied. In the final analysis, it pertains to the conscience either of the sick person, or of those qualified to speak in the sick person's name, or of the doctors, to decide, in the light of moral obligations and of the various aspects of the case.

Everyone has the duty to care for his or her own health or to seek such care from others. Those whose task it is to care for the sick must do so conscientiously and administer the remedies that seem necessary or useful.

However, is it necessary in all circumstances to have recourse to all possible remedies?

In the past, moralists replied that one is never obliged to use "extraordinary" means. This reply, which as a principle still holds good, is perhaps less clear today by reason of the imprecision of the term and the rapid progress made in the treatment of sickness. Thus some people prefer to speak of "proportionate" and "disproportionate" means.

In any case, it will be possible to make a correct judgment as to the means by studying the type of treatment to be used, its degree of complexity or risk, its cost and the possibilities of using it, and comparing these elements with the result that can be expected, taking into account the state of the sick person and his or her physical and moral resources.

In order to facilitate the application of these general principles, the following clarifications can be added:

- If there are no other sufficient remedies, it is permitted, with the patient's consent, to have recourse to the means provided by the most advanced medical techniques, even if these means are still at the experimental stage and are not without a certain risk. By accepting them, the patient can even show generosity in the service of humanity.

- It is also permitted, with the patient's consent, to interrupt these means, where the results fall short of expectations. But for such a decision to be made, account will have to be taken of the reasonable wishes of the patient and the patient's family, as also of the advice of the doctors who are specially competent in the matter. The latter may in particular judge that the investment in instruments and personnel is disproportionate to the results foreseen; they may also judge that the techniques applied impose on the patient strain or suffering out of proportion with the benefits which he or she may gain from such techniques.

- It is also permissible to make do with the normal means that medicine can offer. Therefore one cannot impose on anyone the obligation to have recourse to a technique which is already in use but which carries a risk or is burdensome. Such a refusal is not the equivalent of suicide; on the contrary, it should be considered as an acceptance of the human condition, or a wish to avoid the application of a medical procedure disproportionate to the results that can be expected, or a desire not to impose excessive expense on the family or the community.

- When inevitable death is imminent in spite of the means used, it is permitted in conscience to take the decision to refuse forms of treatment that would only secure a precarious and burdensome prolongation of life, so long as the normal care due to the sick person in similar cases is not interrupted. In such circumstances the doctor has no reason to reproach himself with failing to help the person in danger.

Conclusion

The norms contained in the present Declaration are inspired by a profound desire to service people in accordance with the plan of the Creator. Life is a gift of God, and on the other hand death is unavoidable; it is necessary, therefore, that we, without in any way hastening the hour of death, should be able to accept it with full responsibility and dignity. It is true that death marks the end of our earthly existence, but at the same time it opens the door to immortal life. Therefore, all must prepare themselves for this event in the light of human values, and Christians even more so in the light of faith.

As for those who work in the medical profession, they ought to neglect no means of making all their skill available to the sick and dying; but they should also remember how much more necessary it is to provide them with the comfort of boundless kindness and heartfelt charity. Such service to people is also service to Christ the Lord, who said: "As you did it to one of the least of these my brethren, you did it to me" (Mt. 25:40).

At the audience granted Prefect, His Holiness Pope John Paul II approved this declaration, adopted at the ordinary meeting of the Sacred Congregation for the Doctrine of the Faith, and ordered its publication.

Rome, the Sacred Congregation for the Doctrine of the Faith, May 5, 1980.
Cardinal Franjo Seper
Prefect
Archbishop Jerome Hamer, OP
Secretary

Notes

1. "Declaration on Procured Abortion," November 18, 1974: AAS 66 (1974), pp. 730–47.

2. Pius XII, "Address to those attending the Congress of the International Union of Catholic Women's Leagues," September 11, 1947: *AAS* 39 (1947), p. 483; "Address to Midwives," October 29, 1951: AAS 43 (1951), pp. 835–54; "Speech to the Members of the International Office of Military Medicine Documentation," October 19, 1953: *AAS* 45 (1953), pp. 744–54; "Address to those taking part in the ninth Congress of the Italian Anaesthesiological Society," February 24, 1957: *AAS* 49 (1957), p. 146; cf. also "Address on Re-animation," November 24, 1957: *AAS* 49 (1957), pp. 1027–33; Paul VI, "Address to the Members of the U.N. Special Committee on Apartheid," May 22, 1974: *AAS* 66 (1974), p. 346; John Paul II: "Address to the Bishops of the United States of America," October 5, 1979: *AAS* 71 (1979), p. 1225.

3. One thinks especially of Recommendation 779 (1976) on the rights of the sick and dying, of the Parliamentary Assembly of the Council of Europe at its XXVIIth Ordinary Session; cf. Sipeca, no. 1, March 1977, pp. 14–15.

4. We leave aside completely the problems of the death penalty and of war, which involve specific considerations that do not concern the present subject.

5. Pius XII, "Address" of February 24, 1957: *AAS* 49 (1957), p. 147.

6. Pius XII, ibid., p. 145; cf. "Address" of September 9, 1958: *AAS* 50 (1958), p. 694.

8

The Artificial Prolongation of Life

Pontifical Academy of Sciences

On the invitation of the Pontifical Academy of Sciences, a study group met Oct. 19–21, 1985, to study "the artificial prolongation of life and the exact determination of the moment of death."

After having noted the recent progress of the techniques of resuscitation and the immediate and long-term effects of brain damage, the study group discussed the objective criteria of death and of the rules of conduct in the face of a persistent state of apparent death. On the one hand, experiments carried out reveal that brain resistance to the absence of cerebral circulation can permit recoveries otherwise deemed impossible.

On the other hand, it has been found that when the entire brain has suffered irreversible damage (cerebral death), all possibility of sensitive and cognitive life is definitively ruled out, while a brief vegetative survival can be maintained by artificial prolongation of respiration and circulation.

I. *Definition of Death*

A person is dead when he has irreversibly lost all capacity to integrate and co-ordinate the physical and mental functions of the body.

Death occurs when:

a) The spontaneous cardiac and respiratory functions have definitively ceased; or

b) If an irreversible cessation of every brain function is verified.

From the debate it emerged that cerebral death is the true criterion of death, since the definitive arrest of the cardio-respiratory functions leads very quickly to cerebral death.

The group then analyzed the different clinical and instrumental methods that enable one to ascertain the irreversible arrest of the cerebral functions. To be certain—by means of the electroencephalogram—that the brain has become flat, that is to say, that it no longer displays electric activity, it is necessary that the examination be carried out at least twice at a distance of six hours.

2. Medical Guidelines

By the term treatment the group understands all those medical interventions available and appropriate in a specific case, whatever the complexity of the techniques involved.

If the patient is in a permanent, irreversible coma, as far as can be foreseen, treatment is not required, but all care should be lavished on him, including feeding.

If it is clinically established that there is a possibility of recovery, treatment is required.

If treatment is of no benefit to the patient, it may be interrupted while continuing with the care of the patient.

By the term care the group understands ordinary help due to sick patients, such as compassion and spiritual and affective support due to every human being in danger.

3. Artificial Prolongation of Vegetative Functions

In the case of cerebral death, artificial respiration can prolong the cardiac function for a limited time. This induced survival of the organs is indicated in the case of a foreseen removal of organs for a transplant.

This eventuality is possible only in the case of total and irreversible brain damage occurring in a young person, essentially as a result of a very severe injury.

Taking into consideration the important advances made in surgical techniques and in the means to increase tolerance to transplants, the group holds that transplants deserve the support of the medical profession, of the law and of people in general.

The donation of organs should, in all circumstances, respect the last will of the donor or the consent of the family, if present.

9

On Withdrawing Artificial Nutrition and Hydration

Texas Bishops and the Texas Conference of

Catholic Health Facilities

Human life is God's precious gift to each person. We possess and treasure it as a sacred trust. All persons therefore have a moral responsibility, in accord with their own capacities, roles and personal vocation, to make those decisions and take those necessary steps to preserve and promote their own life and health and that of others. We firmly reiterate the church's continued condemnation of euthanasia as defined in the Vatican's 1980 *Declaration on Euthanasia*.[1]

This responsibility for conserving life and health falls especially upon those persons and institutions directly involved in the healing ministry. Catholic health facilities have a special duty to reflect Roman Catholic teaching while carrying out the compassionate healing ministry of Jesus Christ.

In particular, this commitment to relevant church teaching is exemplified in the treatment of all patients, including those who require life-sustaining procedures. Specifically, the highly controversial issue of the provision of artificial nutrition and hydration is of particular concern today because of the current anti-life ambiance in the United States.

The Texas Conference of Catholic Health Facilities, to ensure consonance with the teachings of the Catholic Church in all of its activities, consulted the bishops of Texas on the subject of forgoing and withdrawing of artificial nutrition and hydration. This consultation contributed to this statement, which addresses the moral aspects of this issue.

Moral Values to Be Promoted and Protected

1. *Human personhood*: Each human person is of incalculable worth because all humans are made in the image of God, redeemed by Christ and are called to share the life of the triune God.

2. *A holistic integration*: This value includes the spiritual, mental, emotional and physical health in the unity of the person and communion of persons. The life and health of the total person and communion of persons are important in order for each person to hear and respond effectively under the influence of grace to God's call.

3. *The inherent sacredness and dignity of the human person*: The life of each person has an inherent dignity, which is to be respected by all other humans. So each person, regardless of age or condition, has exactly the same basic right to life, which deserves equal protection by society and its laws.

Basic Moral Principles

1. *Although life always is a good, there are conditions which, if present, lessen or remove one's obligation to sustain life.* While every reasonable effort should be made to maintain life and restore health, Pope Pius XII noted that there comes a time when these efforts may become excessively burdensome for the patient or others (see Address to International Congress of Anesthesiologists, Nov. 24, 1957).[2]

2. *If the reasonable foreseen benefits to the patient in the use of any means outweigh the burdens to the patient or others, then those means are morally obligatory.* Examples of benefits include cure, pain reduction, restoration of consciousness, restoration of function, and maintenance of life with reasonable hope of recovery. Even without any hope of recovery it is an expression of love and respect for the person to keep the patient clean, warm, and comfortable. There is no moral distinction to be made between the forgoing and withdrawing of life-sustaining procedures.

3. *If the means used to prolong life are disproportionately burdensome compared with the benefits to the patient, then those means need not be used, they are morally optional.*

This principle, taught in the Vatican Declaration on Euthanasia (1980), was built on the teaching of Pope Pius XII and the church's moral tradition.[3] Burdens are those undesirable aspects and consequences of the use of the means themselves which fall upon the patient or others—family, care provider or community. Examples of disproportionate burdens include excessive suffering for the patient; excessive expense for the family or the community; investment in medical technology and personnel disproportionate to the expected results; inequitable resource allocation.[4]

The National Conference of Catholic Bishops' Committee for Pro-Life Activities came to the same conclusion regarding the situation when the burden is disproportionate to the benefits in their statement on the proposed Uniform Rights of the Terminally Ill Act. The statement (July 2, 1986) allowed that "laws dealing with medical treatments may have to take account of exceptional circumstances, where even means for providing nourishment may become too ineffective or burdensome to be obligatory" (*Origins*, July 24, 1986, p. 224).

The *Declaration on Euthanasia*, as well as the teaching of Pius XII, explicitly states that such forgoing or withdrawing are not suicide;[5] rather they should be considered as the acceptance of the human condition and simply letting nature take its course. The omission of life-sustaining means (whether it be a mechanical respirator, a cardiac pacemaker, a renal dialysis machine, or artificial nutrition and hydration) can be acceptable under conditions which render those means morally non-obligatory. In those appropriate cases the decision maker is not guilty of murder, suicide, or assisted suicide, since there is no moral obligation under these circumstances to impede the normal consequences of the underlying pathology. The physical cause of death is ultimately the pathology which required the use of those means in the first place. The proximate physical means are either the absence of the substance necessary for life (oxygen, water, nutrients) or the presence of toxic substances resulting from metabolic activities of the body.

Application to Persistent Vegetative State

Patients, competently diagnosed to be in a persistent vegetative state or in an irreversible coma, remain human persons. Nonetheless, those individuals are stricken with a lethal pathology which, without artificial nutrition and hydration, will lead to death.

The moral issue, then, is what conditions make it morally obligatory to intervene with artificial nutrition and hydration to prevent death, which would otherwise occur as a consequence of the underlying pathology? While each case has to be judged on its own merits, the final decision should be based upon the application of the principles previously described regarding the burden/benefit analysis relative to the use of life-sustaining procedures. Decisions about treatment for unconscious or incompetent patients are to be made by an appropriate proxy (e.g., spouse, parent, adult children) in light of what the patient would have decided. This judgment should be based on the expressed wishes of the patient. The final decision, however, for patients with a fatal pathology, but who are conscious and competent and in the judgment of physicians have no reasonable hope of recovery from it, is to be made by the patients themselves and by no one else.

Patients, even those persons who are in a permanent vegetative state or irreversibly unconscious, should never be abandoned. They should be cared for lovingly—kept clean, warm, and treated with dignity. The morally appropriate forgoing or withdrawing of artificial nutrition and hydration from a permanently unconscious person is not abandoning that person. Rather, it is accepting the fact that the person has come to the end of his or her pilgrimage and should not be impeded from taking the final step. The forgoing or withdrawing of artificial nutrition and hydration should only occur after there has been sufficient deliberation based upon the best medical and personal information available.

Conclusion

The principles are applicable to any life-threatening situation where a person—regardless of age or condition—requires some intervention, especially artificially administered nutrition and hydration, in order to impede the threat to life. In a medical context, the decision needs to be made in each particular case as to whether the normal consequences of a disease or injury should be impeded by human intervention.

All care and treatment should be directed toward the total well-being of the person in need. Because of the high value of temporal health and life, the presumption is made that the necessary steps will be taken to restore health or at least avert death. However, the temporal concerns must always be subordinated to the patient's spiritual needs and obligations.

Catholic health facilities should be particularly sensitive to the pastoral needs of both patients and care givers (family, friends, staff), especially in the context of death and dying.

In the event of doubt about meaning or application of church teaching, the diocesan bishop or his delegate shall be consulted.[6]

Notes

1. "By euthanasia is understood an action or an omission which of itself or by intention causes death, in order that all suffering may in this way be eliminated. Euthanasia's terms of reference, therefore, are to be found in the intention of the will and in the methods used" (*Declaration on Euthanasia*, II).

2. "But normally one is held to use only ordinary means—according to circumstances of persons, places, times, and culture—that is to say, means that don't involve any grave burden for oneself or another. A more strict obligation would be too burdensome for most men and would render the attainment of the higher, more important good too difficult. Life, health, all temporal activities are in fact subordinated to spiritual ends. On the other hand, one is not forbidden to take more than the strictly necessary steps to preserve life and health as long as he does not fail in some more serious duty" (Pope Pius XII, "The Prolongation of Life," Nov. 24, 1957, *The Pope Speaks*, Vol. 4, 1958, pp. 393–98).

3. "In the past, moralists replied that one is never obliged to use 'extraordinary' means. This reply, which as a principle still holds good, is perhaps less clear today, by reason of the imprecision of the term and the rapid progress made in the treatment of sickness. Thus some people prefer to speak of 'proportionate' and 'disproportionate' means" (*Declaration on Euthanasia*, IV, see also n. 4, below).

4. "If there are no other sufficient remedies, it is permitted, with the patient's consent, to have recourse to the means provided by the most advanced medical techniques, even if these means are still at the experimental stage and are not without a certain risk. By accepting them, the patient can even show generosity in the service of humanity.

"It is also permitted, with the patient's consent, to interrupt these means where the results fall short of expectations. But for such a decision to be made, account will have to be taken of the reasonable wishes of the patient's family, as also of the advice of the doctors who are specially competent in the matter. The latter may in particular judge that the investment in instruments and personnel is disproportionate to the results foreseen; they may also judge that the techniques applied impose on the patient strain or suffering out of proportion with the benefits which he or she may gain from such techniques" (ibid.).

5. "It is also permissible to make do with the normal means that medicine can offer. Therefore one cannot impose on anyone the obligation to have recourse to a technique which is already in use but which carries a risk or is burdensome. Such a refusal is not the equivalent of suicide; on the contrary, it should be considered as an acceptance of the human condition, or a wish to avoid the application of a medical procedure disproportionate to the results that can be expected or a desire not to impose excessive expense on the family or the community" (ibid.).

6. The Bishops of Texas are expected to issue a revision of this statement. It can be found at the following website: www.txcatholic.org.

10

Nutrition and Hydration:
Moral and Pastoral Reflections

National Conference of Catholic Bishops' Committee
for Pro-Life Activities

Introduction

Modern medical technology seems to confront us with many questions not
faced even a decade ago. Corresponding changes in medical practice have benefited many but have also prompted fears by some that they will be aggressively
treated against their will or denied the kind of care that is their due as human
persons with inherent dignity. Current debates about life-sustaining treatment
suggest that our society's moral reflection is having difficulty keeping pace with
its technological progress.

A religious view of life has an important contribution to make to these
modern debates. Our Catholic tradition has developed a rich body of thought
on these questions, which affirms a duty to preserve human life but recognizes
limits to that duty.

Our first goal in making this statement is to reaffirm some basic principles
of our moral tradition, to assist Catholics and others in making treatment decisions in accord with respect for God's gift of life.

These principles do not provide clear and final answers to all moral questions that arise as individuals make difficult decisions. Catholic theologians may
differ on how best to apply moral principles to some questions not explicitly
resolved by the Church's teaching authority. Likewise, we understand that those

who must make serious health care decisions for themselves or for others face a complexity of issues, circumstances, thoughts and emotions in each unique case.

This is the case with some questions involving the medically assisted provision of nutrition and hydration to helpless patients—those who are seriously ill, disabled or persistently unconscious. These questions have been made more urgent by widely publicized court cases and the public debate to which they have given rise.

Our second purpose in issuing this statement, then, is to provide some clarification of the moral issues involved in decisions about medically assisted nutrition and hydration. We are fully aware that such guidance is not necessarily final because there are many unresolved medical and ethical questions related to these issues and the continuing development of medical technology will necessitate ongoing reflection. But these decisions already confront patients, families, and health care personnel every day. They arise whenever competent patients make decisions about medically assisted nutrition and hydration for their own present situation, when they consider signing an advance directive such as a "living will" or health care proxy document, and when families or other proxy decision makers make decisions about those entrusted to their care. We offer guidance to those who, facing these issues, might be confused by opinions that at times threaten to deny the inherent dignity of human life. We therefore address our reflections first to those who share our Judeo-Christian traditions, and secondly to others concerned about the dignity and value of human life who seek guidance in making their own moral decisions.

Moral Principles

The Judeo-Christian moral tradition celebrates life as the gift of a loving God, and respects the life of each human being because each is made in the image and likeness of God. As Christians we also believe we are redeemed by Christ and called to share eternal life with Him. From these roots the Catholic tradition has developed a distinctive approach to fostering and sustaining human life. Our Church views life as a sacred trust, a gift over which we are given stewardship and not absolute dominion. The Church thus opposes all direct attacks on innocent life. As conscientious stewards we have a duty to preserve life while recognizing certain limits to that duty:

1. Because human life is the foundation for all other human goods, it has a special value and significance. Life is "the first right of the human person" and "the condition of all the others."[1]

2. All crimes against life, including "euthanasia or willful suicide," must be opposed.[2] Euthanasia is "an action or an omission which of itself or by intention causes death, in order that all suffering may in this way be eliminated." Its terms of reference are to be found "in the intention of the will and in the methods used."[3] Thus defined, euthanasia is an attack on life which no one has a right to make or request, and which no government or other human authority can legitimately recommend or permit. Although individual guilt may be reduced or absent because of suffering or emotional factors that cloud the conscience, this does not change the objective wrongfulness of the act. It should also be recognized that an apparent plea for death may really be a plea for help and love.

3. Suffering is a fact of human life, and has special significance for the Christian as an opportunity to share in Christ's redemptive suffering. Nevertheless there is nothing wrong in trying to relieve someone's suffering; in fact it is a positive good to do so, as long as one does not intentionally cause death or interfere with other moral and religious duties.[4]

4. Everyone has the duty to care for his or her own life and health and to seek necessary medical care from others, but this does not mean that all possible remedies must be used in all circumstances. One is not obliged to use either "extraordinary" means or "disproportionate" means of preserving life—that is, means which are understood as offering no reasonable hope of benefit or as involving excessive burdens. Decisions regarding such means are complex, and should ordinarily be made by the patient in consultation with his or her family, chaplain or pastor, and physician when that is possible.[5]

5. In the final stage of dying one is not obliged to prolong the life of a patient by every possible means: "When inevitable death is imminent in spite of the means used, it is permitted in conscience to take the decision to refuse forms of treatment that would only secure a precarious and burdensome prolongation of life, so long as the normal care due to the sick person in similar cases is not interrupted."[6]

6. While affirming life as a gift of God, the Church recognizes that death is unavoidable and that it can open the door to eternal life. Thus, "without

in any way hastening the hour of death," the dying person should accept its reality and prepare for it emotionally and spiritually.[7]

7. Decisions regarding human life must respect the demands of justice, viewing each human being as our neighbor and avoiding all discrimination based on age or dependency.[8] A human being has "a unique dignity and an independent value, from the moment of conception and in every stage of development, whatever his or her physical condition." In particular, "the disabled person (whether the disability be the result of a congenital handicap, chronic illness or accident, or from mental or physical deficiency, and whatever the severity of the disability) is a fully human subject, with the corresponding innate, sacred, and inviolable rights." First among these is "the fundamental and inalienable right to life."[9]

8. The dignity and value of the human person, which lie at the foundation of the Church's teaching on the right to life, also provide a basis for any just social order. Not only to become more Christian, but to become more truly human, society should protect the right to life through its laws and other policies.[10]

While these principles grow out of a specific religious tradition, they appeal to a common respect for the dignity of the human person. We commend them to all people of good will.

Questions about Medically Assisted Nutrition and Hydration

In what follows we apply these well-established moral principles to the difficult issue of providing medically assisted nutrition and hydration to persons who are seriously ill, disabled, or persistently unconscious. We recognize the complexity involved in applying these principles to individual cases and acknowledge that, at this time and on this particular issue, our applications do not have the same authority as the principles themselves.

1. Is the withholding or withdrawing of medically assisted nutrition and hydration always a direct killing?

In answering this question one should avoid two extremes.

First, it is wrong to say that this could not be a matter of killing simply because it involves an omission rather than a positive action. In fact a deliberate omission may be an effective and certain way to kill, especially to kill someone weakened by illness. Catholic teaching condemns as euthanasia "an action *or an omission* which of itself or by intention causes death, in order that all suffering may in this way be eliminated." Thus "euthanasia includes not only active mercy killing but also the omission of treatment when the purpose of the omission is to kill the patient."[11]

Second, we should not assume that *all or most* decisions to withhold or withdraw medically assisted nutrition and hydration are attempts to cause death. To be sure, any patient will die if all nutrition and hydration are withheld.[12] But sometimes other causes are at work—for example, the patient may be imminently dying, whether feeding takes place or not, from an already existing terminal condition. At other times, although the shortening of the patient's life is one foreseeable result of an omission, the real *purpose* of the omission was to relieve the patient of a particular procedure that was of limited usefulness to the patient or unreasonably burdensome for the patient and the patient's family or caregivers. This kind of decision should not be equated with a decision to kill or with suicide.

The harsh reality is that some who propose withdrawal of nutrition and hydration from certain patients do directly *intend* to bring about a patient's death and would even prefer a change in the law to allow for what they see as more "quick and painless" means to cause death.[13] In other words, nutrition and hydration (whether orally administered or medically assisted) are sometimes withdrawn not because a patient is dying but precisely because a patient is *not* dying (or not dying quickly) and someone believes it would be better if he or she did, generally because the patient is perceived as having an unacceptably low "quality of life" or as imposing burdens on others.[14]

When deciding whether to withhold or withdraw medically assisted nutrition and hydration, or other forms of life support, we are called by our moral tradition to ask ourselves: What will my decision do for this patient? And what am I trying to achieve by doing it? We must be sure that it is not our intent to cause the patient's death—either for its own sake or as a means to achieving some other goal such as the relief of suffering.

2. Is medically assisted nutrition and hydration a form of "treatment" or "care"?

Catholic teaching provides that a person in the final stages of dying need not accept "forms of treatment that would only secure a precarious and burdensome prolongation of life" but should still receive "the normal care due to the sick person in similar cases."[15] All patients deserve to receive normal care out of respect for their inherent dignity as persons. As Pope John Paul II has said, a decision to forgo "purely experimental or ineffective interventions" does not "dispense from the valid therapeutic task of sustaining life or from assistance with the normal means of sustaining life. Science, even when it is unable to heal, can and should care for and assist the sick."[16] But the teaching of the Church has not resolved the question whether medically assisted nutrition and hydration should always be seen as a form of normal care.[17]

Almost everyone agrees that oral feeding, when it can be accepted and assimilated by a patient, is a form of care owed to all helpless people. Christians should be especially sensitive to this obligation because giving food and drink to those in need is an important expression of Christian love and concern (Mt. 10:42 and 25:35; Mk. 9:41). But our obligations become less clear when adequate nutrition and hydration require the skills of trained medical personnel and the use of technologies that may be perceived as very burdensome—that is, as intrusive, painful or repugnant. Such factors vary from one type of feeding procedure to another, and from one patient to another, making it difficult to classify all feeding procedures as either "care" or "treatment."

Perhaps this dilemma should be viewed in a broader context. Even medical "treatments" are morally obligatory when they are "ordinary" means—that is, if they provide a reasonable hope of benefit and do not involve excessive burdens. Therefore we believe people should make decisions in light of a simple and fundamental insight: *Out of respect for the dignity of the human person, we are obliged to preserve our own lives and help others preserve theirs, by the use of means that have a reasonable hope of sustaining life without imposing unreasonable burdens on those we seek to help, that is, on the patient and his or her family and community.*

We must therefore address the question of benefits and burdens next, recognizing that a full moral analysis is only possible when one knows the effects of a given procedure on a particular patient.

3. What are the benefits of medically assisted nutrition and hydration?

According to international codes of medical ethics, a physician will see a medical procedure as appropriate "if in his or her judgment it offers hope of saving life, reestablishing health or alleviating suffering."[18]

Nutrition and hydration, whether provided in the usual way or with medical assistance, do not by themselves remedy pathological conditions, except those caused by dietary deficiencies. But patients benefit from them in several ways. First, for all patients who can assimilate them, suitable food and fluids sustain life, and providing them normally expresses loving concern and solidarity with the helpless. Second, for patients being treated with the hope of a cure, appropriate food and fluids are an important element of sound health care. Third, even for patients who are imminently dying and incurable, food and fluids can prevent the suffering that may arise from dehydration, hunger and thirst.

The benefit of sustaining and fostering life is fundamental because life is our first gift from a loving God and the condition for receiving his other gifts. But sometimes even food and fluids are no longer effective in providing this benefit because a patient has entered the final stage of a terminal condition. At such times we should make the dying person as comfortable as possible and provide nursing care and proper hygiene as well as companionship and appropriate spiritual aid. Such a person may lose all desire for food and drink and even be unable to ingest them. Initiating medically assisted feeding or intravenous fluids in this case may increase the patient's discomfort while providing no real benefit; ice chips or sips of water may instead be appropriate to provide comfort and counteract the adverse effects of dehydration.[19] Even in the case of the imminently dying patient, of course, any action or omission that of itself or by intention causes death is to be absolutely rejected.

As Christians who trust in the promise of eternal life, we recognize that death does not have the final word. Accordingly we need not always prevent death until the last possible moment; but we should never intentionally cause death or abandon the dying person as though he or she were unworthy of care and respect.

4. What are the burdens of medically assisted nutrition and hydration?

Our tradition does not demand heroic measures in fulfilling the obligation to sustain life. A person may legitimately refuse even procedures that effectively prolong life, if he or she believes they would impose excessively grave burdens on himself or herself, or on his or her family and community. Catholic theologians have traditionally viewed medical treatment as excessively burdensome if it is "too painful, too damaging to the patient's bodily self and functioning, too psychologically repugnant to the patient, too restrictive of the patient's liberty and preferred activities, too suppressive of the patient's mental life, or too expensive."[20]

Because assessment of these burdens necessarily involves some subjective judgments, a conscious and competent patient is generally the best judge of whether a particular burden or risk is too grave to be tolerated in his or her own case. But because of the serious consequences of withdrawing all nutrition and hydration, patients and those helping them make decisions should assess such burdens or risks with special care.

Here we offer some brief reflections and cautions regarding the kinds of burdens sometimes associated with medically assisted nutrition and hydration.

PHYSICAL RISKS AND BURDENS

The risks and objective complications of medically assisted nutrition and hydration will depend on the procedure used and the condition of the patient. In a given case a feeding procedure may become harmful or even life-threatening. (These medical data are discussed at length in an Appendix to this paper.)

If the risks and burdens of a particular feeding procedure are deemed serious enough to warrant withdrawing it, we should not automatically deprive the patient of all nutrition and hydration but should ask whether another procedure is feasible that would be less burdensome. We say this because some helpless patients, including some in a "persistent vegetative state," receive tube feedings not because they cannot swallow food at all but because tube feeding is less costly and difficult for health care personnel.[21]

Moreover, because burdens are assessed in relation to benefits, we should ask whether the risks and discomfort of a feeding procedure are really excessive as compared with the adverse effects of dehydration or malnutrition.

PSYCHOLOGICAL BURDENS ON THE PATIENT

Many people see feeding tubes as frightening or even as bodily violations. Assessments of such burdens are necessarily subjective; they should not be dismissed on that account, but we offer some practical cautions to help prevent abuse.

First, in keeping with our moral teaching against the intentional causing of death by omission, one should distinguish between repugnance to a particular procedure and repugnance to life itself. The latter may occur when a patient views a life of helplessness and dependency on others as itself a heavy burden, leading him or her to wish or even to pray for death. Especially in our achievement-oriented society, the burden of living in such a condition may seem to outweigh any possible benefit of medical treatment and even lead a person to despair. But we should not assume that the burdens in such a case always outweigh the benefits; for the sufferer, given good counseling and spiritual support, may be brought again to appreciate the precious gift of life.

Second, our tradition recognizes that when treatment decisions are made, "account will have to be taken of the *reasonable* wishes of the patient and the patient's family, as also of the advice of the doctors who are specially competent in the matter."[22] The word "reasonable" is important here. Good health care providers will try to help patients assess psychological burdens with full information and without undue fear of unfamiliar procedures.[23] A well-trained and compassionate hospital chaplain can provide valuable personal and spiritual support to patients and families facing these difficult situations.

Third, we should not assume that a feeding procedure is inherently repugnant to all patients without specific evidence. In contrast to Americans' general distaste for the idea of being supported by "tubes and machines," some studies indicate surprisingly favorable views of medically assisted nutrition and hydration among patients and families with actual experience of such procedures.[24]

ECONOMIC AND OTHER BURDENS ON CAREGIVERS

While some balk at the idea, in principle cost can be a valid factor in decisions about life support. For example, money spent on expensive treatment for one family member may be money otherwise needed for food, housing, and other necessities for the rest of the family. Here, also, we offer some cautions.

First, particularly when a form of treatment "carries a risk or is burdensome" on other grounds, a critically ill person may have a legitimate and altruistic desire "not to impose excessive expense on the family or the community."[25] Even for altruistic reasons a patient should not directly intend his or her own death by malnutrition or dehydration, but may accept an earlier death as a consequence of his or her refusal of an unreasonably expensive treatment. Decisions *by others* to deny an incompetent patient medically assisted nutrition and hydration for reasons of cost raise additional concerns about justice to the individual patient, who could wrongly be deprived of life itself to serve the less fundamental needs of others.

Second, we do not think individual decisions about medically assisted nutrition and hydration should be determined by macro-economic concerns such as national budget priorities and the high cost of health care. These social problems are serious, but it is by no means established that they require depriving chronically ill and helpless patients of effective and easily tolerated measures that they need to survive.[26]

Third, a tube feeding alone is generally not very expensive and may cost no more than oral feeding.[27] What is seen by many as a grave financial and emotional burden on caregivers is the total long-term care of severely debilitated patients, who may survive for many years with no life support except medically assisted nutrition and hydration and nursing care.

The difficulties families may face in this regard, and their need for improved financial and other assistance from the rest of society, should not be underestimated. While caring for a helpless loved one can provide many intangible benefits to family members and bring them closer together, the responsibilities of care can also strain even close and loving family relationships; complex medical decisions must be made under emotionally difficult circumstances not easily appreciated by those who have never faced such situations.

Even here, however, we must try to think through carefully what we intend by withdrawing medically assisted nutrition and hydration. Are we deliberately trying to make sure that the patient dies, in order to relieve caregivers of the financial and emotional burdens that will fall upon them if the patient survives? Are we really implementing a decision to withdraw all other forms of care, precisely because the patient offers so little response to the efforts of caregivers? Decisions like these seem to reach beyond the weighing of burdens and benefits of medically assisted nutrition and hydration as such.

In the context of official Church teaching, it is not yet clear to what extent we may assess the burden of a patient's total care rather than the burden of a particular treatment when we seek to refuse "burdensome" life support. On a practical level, those seeking to make good decisions might assure themselves of their own intentions by asking: Does my decision aim at relieving the patient of a particularly grave burden imposed by medically assisted nutrition and hydration? Or does it aim to avoid the total burden of caring for the patient? If so, does it achieve this aim by deliberately bringing about his or her death?

Rather than leaving families to confront such dilemmas alone, society and government should improve their assistance to families whose financial and emotional resources are strained by long-term care of loved ones.[28]

5. What role should "quality of life" play in our decisions?

Financial and emotional burdens are willingly endured by most families to raise their children or to care for mentally aware but weak and elderly family members. It is sometimes argued that we need not endure comparable burdens to feed and care for persons with severe mental and physical disabilities, because their low "quality of life" makes it unnecessary or pointless to preserve their lives.[29]

But this argument—even when it seems motivated by a humanitarian concern to reduce suffering and hardship—ignores the equal dignity and sanctity of all human life. Its key assumption—that people with disabilities necessarily enjoy life less than others or lack the potential to lead meaningful lives—is also mistaken.[30] Where suffering does exist, society's response should not be to neglect or eliminate the lives of people with disabilities, but to help correct their inadequate living conditions.[31] Very often the worst threat to a good "quality of life" for these people is not the disability itself but the prejudicial attitudes of others—attitudes based on the idea that a life with serious disabilities is not worth living.[32]

This being said, our moral tradition allows for three ways in which the "quality of life" of a seriously ill patient is relevant to treatment decisions:

1. Consistent with respect for the inherent sanctity of life, we should relieve needless suffering and support morally acceptable ways of improving each patient's quality of life.[33]

2. One may legitimately refuse a treatment because it would itself create an impairment imposing *new* serious burdens or risks on the patient. This decision to avoid the new burdens or risks created by a treatment is not the same as directly intending to end life in order to avoid the burden of living in a disabled state.[34]

3. Sometimes a disabling condition may directly influence the benefits and burdens of a specific treatment for a particular patient. For example, a confused or demented patient may find medically assisted nutrition and hydration more frightening and burdensome than other patients do because he or she cannot understand what it is. The patient may even repeatedly pull out feeding tubes, requiring burdensome physical restraints if this form of feeding is to be continued. In such cases, ways of alleviating such special burdens should be explored before concluding that they justify withholding all food and fluids needed to sustain life.

These humane considerations are quite different from a "quality of life" ethic that would judge individuals with disabilities or limited potential as not worthy of care or respect. It is one thing to withhold a procedure because it would impose new disabilities on a patient, and quite another thing to say that patients who already have such disabilities should not have their lives preserved.

A means considered ordinary or proportionate for other patients should not be considered extraordinary or disproportionate for severely impaired patients solely because of a judgment that their lives are not worth living.

In short, while considerations regarding a person's quality of life have some validity in weighing the burdens and benefits of medical treatment, at the present time in our society judgments about the quality of life are sometimes used to promote euthanasia. The Church must emphasize the sanctity of life of each person as a fundamental principle in all moral decision making.

6. Do persistently unconscious patients represent a special case?

Even Catholics who accept the same basic moral principles may strongly disagree on how to apply them to patients who appear to be persistently unconscious—that is, those who are in a permanent coma or a "persistent vegetative state" (PVS).[35] Some moral questions in this area have not been explicitly resolved by the Church's teaching authority.

On some points there is wide agreement among Catholic theologians:

1. An unconscious patient must be treated as a living human person with inherent dignity and value. Direct killing of such a patient is as morally reprehensible as the direct killing of anyone else. Even the medical terminology used to describe these patients as "vegetative" unfortunately tends to obscure this vitally important point, inviting speculation that a patient in this state is a "vegetable" or a subhuman animal.[36]

2. The area of legitimate controversy does not concern patients with conditions like mental retardation, senility, dementia or even temporary unconsciousness. Where serious disagreement begins is with the patient who has been diagnosed as completely and permanently unconscious after careful testing over a period of weeks or months.

Some moral theologians argue that a particular form of care or treatment is morally obligatory only when its benefits outweigh its burdens to a patient or the care providers. In weighing burdens, they say, the total burden of a procedure and the consequent requirements of care must be taken into account. If no benefit can be demonstrated, the procedure, whatever its burdens, cannot be obligatory. These moralists also hold that the chief criterion to determine the benefit of a procedure cannot be merely that it prolongs physical life, since physical life is not an absolute good but is relative to the spiritual good of the person. They assert that the spiritual good of the person is union with God, which can be advanced only by human acts, i.e., conscious, free acts. Since the best current medical opinion holds that persons in the persistent vegetative state (PVS) are incapable now or in the future of conscious, free human acts, these moralists conclude that, when careful diagnosis verifies this condition, it is not obligatory to prolong life by such interventions as a respirator, antibiotics, or medically assisted hydration and nutrition. To decide to omit non-obligatory care, therefore, is not to intend the patient's death but only to avoid the burden of the procedure. Hence, though foreseen, the patient's death is to be attributed to the patient's pathological condition and not to the omission of care. Therefore, these theologians conclude, while it is always wrong directly to intend or cause the death of such patients, the natural dying process which would have occurred without these interventions may be permitted to proceed.

While this rationale is convincing to some, it is not theologically conclusive and we are not persuaded by it. In fact, other theologians argue cogently that theological inquiry could lead one to a more carefully limited conclusion.

These moral theologians argue that while particular treatments can be judged useless or burdensome, it is morally questionable and would create a dangerous precedent to imply that any human life is not a positive good or "benefit." They emphasize that while life is not the highest good, it is always and everywhere a basic good of the human person and not merely a means to other goods. They further assert that if the "burden" one is trying to relieve by discontinuing medically assisted nutrition and hydration is the burden of remaining alive in the allegedly undignified condition of PVS, such a decision is unacceptable, because one's intent is only achieved by deliberately ensuring the patient's death from malnutrition or dehydration. Finally, these moralists suggest that PVS is best seen as an extreme form of mental and physical disability—one whose causes, nature and prognosis are as yet imperfectly understood—and not as a terminal illness or fatal pathology from which patients should generally be allowed to die. Because the patient's life can often be sustained indefinitely by medically assisted nutrition and hydration that is not unreasonably risky or burdensome for that patient, they say, we are not dealing here with a case where "inevitable death is imminent in spite of the means used."[37] Rather, because the patient will die in a few days if medically assisted nutrition and hydration are discontinued,[38] but can often live a long time if they are provided, the inherent dignity and worth of the human person obligates us to provide this patient with care and support.

Further complicating this debate is a disagreement over what responsible Catholics should do in the absence of a final resolution of this question. Some point to our moral tradition of probabilism, which would allow individuals to follow the appropriate moral analysis that they find persuasive. Others point to the principle that in cases where one might risk unjustly depriving someone of life, we should take the safer course.

In the face of the uncertainties and unresolved medical and theological issues, it is important to defend and preserve important values. On the one hand, there is a concern that patients and families should not be subjected to unnecessary burdens, ineffective treatments and indignities when death is approaching. On the other hand, it is important to ensure that the inherent dignity of human persons, even those who are persistently unconscious, is respected and that no one is deprived of nutrition and hydration with the intent of bringing on his or her death.

It is not easy to arrive at a single answer to some of the real and personal dilemmas involved in this issue. In study, prayer and compassion we continue to reflect on this issue and hope to discover additional information that will lead to its ultimate resolution.

In the meantime, at a practical level, we are concerned that withdrawal of all life support, including nutrition and hydration, not be viewed as appropriate or automatically indicated for the entire class of PVS patients simply because of a judgment that they are beyond the reach of medical treatment that would restore consciousness. We note the current absence of conclusive scientific data on the causes and implications of different degrees of brain damage, on the PVS patient's ability to experience pain, and on the reliability of prognoses for many such patients.[39] We do know that many of these patients have a good prognosis for long-term survival when given medically assisted nutrition and hydration, and a certain prognosis for death otherwise—and we know that many in our society view such an early death as a positive good for a patient in this condition. Therefore we are gravely concerned about current attitudes and policy trends in our society that would too easily dismiss patients without apparent mental faculties as non-persons or as undeserving of human care and concern. In this climate, even legitimate moral arguments intended to have a careful and limited application can easily be misinterpreted, broadened and abused by others to erode respect for the lives of some of our society's most helpless members.

In light of these concerns, it is our considered judgment that while legitimate Catholic moral debate continues, decisions about these patients should be guided by a presumption in favor of medically assisted nutrition and hydration. A decision to discontinue such measures should be made in light of a careful assessment of the burdens and benefits of nutrition and hydration for the individual patient and his or her family and community. Such measures must not be withdrawn in order to cause death, but they may be withdrawn if they offer no reasonable hope of sustaining life or pose excessive risks or burdens. We also believe that social and health care policies should be carefully framed so that these patients are not routinely classified as "terminal" or as prime candidates for the discontinuance of even minimal means of life support.

7. *Who should make decisions about medically assisted nutrition and hydration?*

"Who decides?" In our society many believe this is the most important or even the only important question regarding this issue; and many understand it in terms of who has *legal* status to decide. Our Catholic tradition is more concerned with the principles for good *moral* decision making, which apply to everyone involved in a decision. Some general observations are appropriate here.

A competent patient is the primary decision maker about his or her own health care, and is in the best situation to judge how the benefits and burdens of a particular procedure will be experienced. Ideally the patient will act with the advice of loved ones, of health care personnel who have expert knowledge of medical aspects of the case, and of pastoral counselors who can help explore the moral issues and spiritual values involved. A patient may wish to make known his or her general wishes about life support in advance; such expressions cannot have the weight of a fully informed decision made in the actual circumstances of an illness, but can help guide others in the event of a later state of incompetency.[40] Morally even the patient making decisions for himself or herself is bound by norms that prohibit the directly intended causing of death through action or omission, and by the distinction between ordinary and extraordinary means.

When a patient is not competent to make his or her own decisions, a proxy decision maker who shares the patient's moral convictions, such as a family member or guardian, may be designated to represent the patient's interests and interpret his or her wishes. Here, too, moral limits remain relevant—that is, morally the proxy may not deliberately cause a patient's death or refuse what is clearly ordinary means, even if he or she believes the patient would have made such a decision.

Health care personnel should generally follow the reasonable wishes of patient or family, but must also consult their own consciences when participating in these decisions. A physician or nurse told to participate in a course of action that he or she views as clearly immoral has a right and responsibility either to refuse to participate in this course of action or to withdraw from the case, and he or she should be given the opportunity to express the reasons for such refusal in the appropriate forum. Social and legal policies must protect such rights of conscience.

Finally, because these are matters of life and death for human persons, society as a whole has a legitimate interest in responsible decision making.[41]

Conclusion

In this document we reaffirm moral principles that provide a basis for responsible discussion of the morality of life support. We also offer tentative guidance on how to apply these principles to the difficult issue of medically assisted nutrition and hydration.

We reject any omission of nutrition and hydration intended to cause a patient's death. We hold for a presumption in favor of providing medically assisted nutrition and hydration to patients who need it, which presumption would yield in cases where such procedures have no medically reasonable hope of sustaining life or pose excessive risks or burdens. Recognizing that judgments about the benefits and burdens of medically assisted nutrition and hydration in individual cases have a subjective element and are generally best made by the patient directly involved, we also affirm a legitimate role for families' love and guidance, health care professionals' ethical concerns, and society's interest in preserving life and protecting the helpless. In rejecting broadly permissive policies on withdrawal of nutrition and hydration from vulnerable patients, we must also help ensure that the burdens of caring for the helpless are more equitably shared throughout our society.

We recognize that this document is our first word, not our last word, on some of the complex questions involved in this subject. We urge Catholics and others concerned about the dignity of the human person to study these reflections and participate in the continuing public discussion of how best to address the needs of the helpless in our society.

Appendix
Technical Aspects of Medically Assisted
Nutrition and Hydration

Procedures for providing nourishment and fluids to patients who cannot swallow food orally are either "parenteral" (bypassing the digestive tract) or "enteral" (using the digestive tract).

Parenteral or intravenous feeding is generally considered "more hazardous and more expensive" than enteral feeding.[42] It can be subdivided into peripheral intravenous feeding (using a needle inserted into a peripheral vein) and central intravenous feeding, also known as total parenteral feeding or hyperalimentation (using a larger needle inserted into a central vein near the heart). Peripheral intravenous lines can provide fluids and electrolytes as well as some nutrients; they can maintain fluid balance and prevent dehydration, but cannot provide adequate nutrition in the long term.[43] Total parenteral feeding can provide a more adequate nutritional balance but poses significant risks to the patient and may involve costs an order of magnitude higher than other methods of tube feeding. It is no longer considered experimental, and has become "a mainstay for helping critically ill patients to survive acute illnesses where the prognosis had previously been nearly hopeless," but its feasibility for life-long maintenance of patients without a functioning gastrointestinal tract has been questioned.[44]

Because of the limited usefulness of peripheral intravenous feeding and the special burdens of total parenteral feeding—and because few patients so completely lack a digestive system that they must depend on these measures for their sole source of nutrition—enteral tube feeding is the focus of the current debate over medically assisted nutrition and hydration. Such methods are used when a patient has a functioning digestive system but is unable or unwilling to ingest food orally and/or to swallow. The most common routes for enteral tube feeding are nasogastric (introducing a thin plastic tube through the nasal cavity to reach into the stomach), gastrostomy (surgical insertion of a tube through the abdominal wall into the stomach), and jejunostomy (surgical insertion of a tube through the abdominal wall into the small intestine).[45] These methods are the primary focus of this document.

Each method of enteral tube feeding has potential side effects. For example, nasogastric tubes must be inserted and monitored carefully so they will not introduce food or fluids into the lungs. They may also irritate sensitive tissues and create discomfort; confused or angry patients may sometimes try to remove them, and efforts to restrain a patient to prevent this can impose additional discomfort and other burdens. On the positive side, insertion of these tubes requires no surgery and only a modicum of training.[46]

Gastrostomy and jejunostomy tubes are better tolerated by many patients in need of long-term feeding. Their most serious physical burdens arise from the fact that their insertion requires surgery using local or general anesthesia, which involves some risk of infection and other complications. Once the surgical procedure is completed, these tubes can often be maintained without serious pain or medical complications, and confused patients do not often attempt to remove them.[47]

Notes

1. Congregation for the Doctrine of the Faith, *Declaration on Procured Abortion* (1974), no. 11.

2. Second Vatican Council, *Gaudium et spes*, no. 27. Suicide must be distinguished from "that sacrifice of one's life whereby for a higher cause, such as God's glory, the salvation of souls or the higher service of one's brethren, a person offers his or her own life or puts it in danger." Congregation for the Doctrine of the Faith, *Declaration on Euthanasia* (1980), Part I.

3. *Declaration on Euthanasia*, Part II.

4. See: *Declaration on Euthanasia*, Part III; United States Catholic Conference, *Ethical and Religious Directives for Catholic Health Facilities* (1971), Directive 29.

5. *Declaration on Euthanasia*, Part IV.

6. *Declaration on Euthanasia*, Part IV.

7. *Declaration on Euthanasia*, Conclusion.

8. *Gaudium et spes*, no. 27; *Declaration on Procured Abortion*, no. 12.

9. *Document of the Holy See for the International Year of Disabled Persons* (March 4, 1981), I.1 and II.1: *Origins*, Vol. 10 (1981), pp. 747–48.

10. *Declaration on Euthanasia*, Introduction; *Declaration on Procured Abortion*, nos. 10–11, 21; Sacred Congregation for the Doctrine of the Faith, *Instruction on Respect for Human Life in Its Origin* (1987), Part III.

11. Archbishop John Roach, "Life-support removal: No easy answers," *Catholic Bulletin*, March 7, 1991, p. 1 (citing Bio/medical Ethics Commission of the Archdiocese of St. Paul-Minneapolis).

12. "If all fluids and nutrition are withdrawn from any patient, regardless of the condition, he or she will die—inevitably and invariably. Death may come in a few days or take up to two weeks. Rarely in medicine is an earlier death for the patient so certain." Ronald E. Cranford, MD, "Patients with Permanent Loss of Consciousness," in Joanne Lynn (ed.), *By No Extraordinary Means* (Indiana University Press 1986), p. 191.

13. See the arguments made by a judge in the Elizabeth Bouvia case, and by attorneys in the Hector Rodas case, among others. See *Bouvia v. Superior Court*, 225 Cal. Rptr. 297, 307–8 (1986) (Compton, J., concurring); *Complaint for Declaratory Relief in Rodas Case, Issues in Law & Medicine*, Vol. 2 (1987), pp. 499–501, quoted verbatim from *Rodas v. Erkenbrack*, No. 87 ev 142 (Mesa County, Colo., filed Jan. 30, 1987).

14. As one medical ethicist observes, interest in a broadly permissive policy for removing nutrition and hydration has grown "because a denial of nutrition may in the long run become the only effective way to make certain that a large number of biologically tenacious patients actually die." Daniel Callahan, "On Feeding the Dying," *Hastings Center Report*, Vol. 13 (October 1983), p. 22.

15. See "Moral Principles" above, no. 5.

16. Address to a Human Pre-Leukaemia Conference, November 15, 1985: *AAS*, Vol.78 (1986), p. 361. Also see his October 21, 1985 address to a study group of the Pontifical Academy of Sciences: "Even when the sick are incurable they are never untreatable; whatever their condition, appropriate care should be provided for them." *AAS*, Vol. 78 (1986), p. 314; *Origins*, Vol. 15 (December 5, 1985), p. 416.

17. Some groups advising the Holy See have ventured opinions on this point, but these do not have the force of official Church teaching. For example, in 1985 a study group of the Pontifical Academy of Sciences concluded: "If the patient is in a permanent, irreversible coma, as far as can be foreseen, treatment is not required, but all care should be lavished on him, including feeding." Pontifical Academy of Sciences, "The Artificial Prolongation of Life," *Origins*, Vol. 15 (December 5, 1985), p. 415. Since comatose patients cannot generally take food orally, the statement evidently refers to medically assisted feeding. Similar statements are found in: Pontifical Council Cor Unum, *Question of Ethics Regarding the Fatally Ill and the Dying* (1981), p. 9; "Ne Eutanasia Ne Accanimento Terapeutico," *La Civilta Cattolica*, Vol. 3280 (February 21, 1987), p. 324.

18. World Medical Association, *Declaration of Helsinki* (1975), II.1.

19. See Joyce V. Zerwekh, "The Dehydration Question," *Nursing 83* (January 1983), pp. 47–51.

20. See William E. May, et al., "Feeding and Hydrating the Permanently Unconscious and Other Vulnerable Persons," *Issues in Law and Medicine*, Vol. 2 (Winter 1987), p. 208.

21. Ronald E. Cranford, "The Persistent Vegetative State: The Medical Reality (Getting the Facts Straight)," *Hastings Center Report*, Vol. 18 (February/March 1988), p. 31.

22. *Declaration on Euthanasia*, Part IV (emphasis added).

23. Current ethical guidelines for nurses, while generally defending patient autonomy, reflect this concern: "Obligations to prevent harm and bring benefit . . . require that nurses seek to understand the patient's reasons for refusal. . . . Nurses should make every effort to correct inaccurate views, to modify superficially held beliefs and overly dramatic gestures, and to restore hope where there is reason to hope." American Nurses' Association Committee on Ethics, "Guidelines on Withdrawing or Withholding Food and Fluid," *Biolaw*, Vol. 2 (October 1988), pp. U1124–25.

24. In one such study, "70 percent of patients and families were 100 percent willing to undergo intensive care again to achieve even one month of survival"; "age, severity of critical illness, length of stay, and charges for intensive care did not influence willingness to undergo intensive care." Danis, et al., "Patients' and Families' Preferences for Medical Intensive Care," *Journal of the*

American Medical Association, Vol. 260 (Aug. 12, 1988), p. 797. In another study, out of 33 people who had close relatives in a "persistent vegetative state," 29 agreed with the initial decision to initiate tube feeding and 25 strongly agreed that such feeding should be continued, although none of those surveyed had made the decision to initiate it. Tresch, et al., "Patients in a Persistent Vegetative State: Attitudes and Reactions of Family Members," *Journal of the American Geriatrics Society*, Vol. 39 (January 1991), pp. 17–21.

25. *Declaration on Euthanasia*, Part IV.

26. "In striving to contain medical care costs, it is important to avoid discriminating against the critically ill and dying, to shun invidious comparisons of the economic value of various individuals to society, and to refuse to abandon patients and hasten death to save money." Hastings Center, *Guidelines on the Termination of Life Sustaining Treatment and the Care of the Dying* (Hastings Center 1987), p. 120.

27. A possible exception is total parenteral feeding, which requires carefully prepared sterile formulas and more intensive daily monitoring. Ironically, some current health care policies may exert economic pressure in favor of TPN because it is easier to obtain third-party reimbursement. Families may pay more for other forms of feeding because some insurance companies do *not* see them as "medical treatment." See U.S. Congress, Office of Technology Assessment, *Life-Sustaining Technologies and the Elderly*, OTA-BA-306 (Washington, D.C.: July 1987), p. 286.

28. "One can never claim that one wishes to bring comfort to a family by suppressing one of its members. The respect, the dedication, the time and means required for the care of handicapped persons, even of those whose mental faculties are gravely affected, is the price that a society should generously pay in order to remain truly human." *Document of the Holy See*, note 9 *supra*, II.I: *Origins*, p. 748. The Holy See acknowledges that society as a whole should willingly assume these burdens, not leave them on the shoulders of individuals and families.

29. E.g., see P. Singer, "Sanctity of Life or Quality of Life?," *Pediatrics*, Vol. 72 (July 1983), pp. 128–29. On the use and misuse of the term "quality of life" see John Cardinal O'Connor, "Who Will Care for the AIDS Victims?," *Origins*, Vol. 19 (January 18, 1990), pp. 544–48. Some Catholic theologians argue that a low "quality of life" justifies withdrawal of medically assisted feeding only from patients diagnosed as permanently unconscious. This argument is discussed separately in section 6 below.

30. See David Milne, "Urges MDs to Get Birth Defects Patient's Own Story," *Medical Tribune* (December 12, 1979), p. 6.

31. National Conference of Catholic Bishops, *Pastoral Statement of the United States Catholic Bishops on Persons with Disabilities* (Washington, D.C.: USCC 1978).

32. Some patients with disabilities ask for death because all their efforts to build a life of self-respect are thwarted; a "right to die" is the first right for which they receive enthusiastic support from the able-bodied. See Paul K. Longmore, "Elizabeth Bouvia, Assisted Suicide and Social Prejudice," *Issues in Law & Medicine*, Vol. 3 (Fall 1987), pp. 141–68.

33. "Quality of life must be sought, in so far as it is possible, by proportionate and appropriate treatment, but it presupposes life and the right to life for everyone, without discrimination and abandonment." Pope John Paul II, Address of April 14, 1988, to the Eleventh European Congress of Perinatal Medicine: *AAS*, Vol. 80 (1988), p. 1426; *The Pope Speaks*, Vol. 33 (1988), pp. 264–65.

34. See Archbishop Roger Mahony, "Two Statements on the Bouvia Case," *Linacre Quarterly*, Vol. 55 (February 1988), pp. 85–87.

35. Coma and persistent vegetative state are not the same. Coma, strictly speaking, is generally not a long-term condition, for within a few weeks a comatose patient usually dies, recovers, or reaches the plateau of a persistent vegetative state. "*Coma* implies the absence of both arousal and content. In terms of observable behavior, the comatose patient appears to be asleep, but unlike the sleeping patient, he cannot be aroused from this state. . . . The patient in the vegetative state appears awake but shows no evidence of content, either confused or appropriate. He often has sleep-wake cycles but cannot demonstrate an awareness of himself or his environment." Levy, "The Comatose Patient," in Rosenberg (ed.), *The Clinical Neurosciences* (Churchill Livingstone 1983), Vol. I, p. 956.

36. While this pejorative connotation was surely not intended by those coining the phrase, we invite the medical profession to consider a less discriminatory term for this diagnostic state.

37. See "Moral Principles" above, n. 5.

38. Because patients need nutritional support to live during the weeks and months of observation required for a responsible assessment of PVS, the cases discussed here involve decisions about discontinuing such support rather than initiating it.

39. One recent scientific study of recovery rates followed up eighty-four patients with a firm diagnosis of PVS. Of these patients, "41 percent became conscious by six months, 52 percent regained consciousness by one year and 58 percent recovered consciousness within the three-year follow-up interval." The study was unable to identify "predictors of recovery from the vegetative state"—that is, there is no established test by which physicians can tell in advance which PVS patients will ultimately wake up. The data "do not exclude the possibility of vegetative patients regaining consciousness after the second year," though this "must be regarded as a rare event." Levin, Saydja, et al., "Vegetative State after Closed-Head Injury: A Traumatic Coma Data Bank Report," *Archives of Neurology*, Vol. 48 (June 1991), pp. 580–85.

40. Some Catholic moralists, using the concept of a "virtual intention," note that a person may give spiritual significance to his or her later suffering during incompetency, by deciding in advance to join these sufferings with those of Christ for the redemption of others.

41. See: NCCB Committee for Pro-Life Activities, "Guidelines for Legislation on Life Sustaining Treatment" (November 10, 1984), *Origins*, Vol. 14 (January 24, 1985); "Statement on the Uniform Rights of the Terminally Ill Act" (June 1986), *Origins*, Vol. 16 (September 4, 1986); United States Catholic Conference, Brief as Amicus Curiae in Support of Petitioners, *Cruzan v. Director of Missouri Department of Health v. McCanse*, U.S. Supreme Court, No. 88-1503, *Origins*, Vol. 19 (October 26, 1989), pp. 345–51.

42. David Major, MD, "The Medical Procedures for Providing Food and Water: Indications and Effects," in Lynn (ed.), *By No Extraordinary Means* (Indiana University Press 1986) [hereinafter "Major"], p. 27.

43. Peripheral veins (e.g., those found in an arm or leg) will eventually collapse after a period of intravenous feeding, and will collapse much faster if complex nutrients such as proteins are included in the formula. See U.S. Congress, Office of Technology Assessment, *Life-Sustaining Technologies and the Elderly*, OTA-BA-306 (Washington, D.C.: U.S. Government Printing Office, July 1987) [hereinafter "OTA"], pp. 283–84.

44. Major, pp. 22, 24–25. Also see OTA, pp. 284–86.

45. See Major, pp. 22, 25–26.

46. Major, p. 22; OTA, pp. 282-3; Ross Laboratories, *Tube Feedings: Clinical Application* (1982), pp. 28–30.

47. Major, p. 22; OTA, p. 282. Many ethicists observe that there is no morally significant difference in principle between withdrawing a life-sustaining procedure and failing to initiate it. However, surgically implanting a feeding tube and maintaining it once implanted may involve a different proportion of benefit to burden, because the transient risks of the initial surgical procedure will not continue or recur during routine maintenance of the tube.

11

Ethical and Religious Directives:
Introduction to Part V and Directives 57–58

United States Conference of Catholic Bishops

PART 5

Issues in Care for the Dying

INTRODUCTION

Christ's redemption and saving grace embrace the whole person, especially in his or her illness, suffering, and death.[35] The Catholic health care ministry faces the reality of death with the confidence of faith. In the face of death—for many, a time when hope seems lost—the Church witnesses to her belief that God has created each person for eternal life.[36]

Above all, as a witness to its faith, a Catholic health care institution will be a community of respect, love, and support to patients or residents and their families as they face the reality of death. What is hardest to face is the process of dying itself, especially the dependency, the helplessness, and the pain that so often accompany terminal illness. One of the primary purposes of medicine in caring for the dying is the relief of pain and the suffering caused by it. Effective management of pain in all its forms is critical in the appropriate care of the dying.

The truth that life is a precious gift from God has profound implications for the question of stewardship over human life. We are not the owners of our lives and, hence, do not have absolute power over life. We have a duty to preserve our life and to use it for the glory of God, but the duty to preserve life is not absolute, for we may reject life-prolonging procedures that are insufficiently beneficial or excessively burdensome. Suicide and euthanasia are never morally acceptable options.

The task of medicine is to care even when it cannot cure. Physicians and their patients must evaluate the use of the technology at their disposal. Reflection on the innate dignity of human life in all its dimensions and on the purpose of medical care is indispensable for formulating a true moral judgment about the use of technology to maintain life. The use of life-sustaining technology is judged in light of the Christian meaning of life, suffering, and death. Only in this way are two extremes avoided: on the one hand, an insistence on useless or burdensome technology even when a patient may legitimately wish to forgo it and, on the other hand, the withdrawal of technology with the intention of causing death.[37]

Some state Catholic conferences, individual bishops, and the USCCB Committee on Pro-Life Activities (formerly an NCCB committee) have addressed the moral issues concerning medically assisted hydration and nutrition. The bishops are guided by the Church's teaching forbidding euthanasia, which is "an action or an omission which of itself or by intention causes death, in order that all suffering may in this way be eliminated."[38] These statements agree that hydration and nutrition are not morally obligatory either when they bring no comfort to a person who is imminently dying or when they cannot be assimilated by a person's body. The USCCB Committee on Pro-Life Activities' report, in addition, points out the necessary distinctions between questions already resolved by the magisterium and those requiring further reflection, as, for example, the morality of withdrawing medically assisted hydration and nutrition from a person who is in the condition that is recognized by physicians as the "persistent vegetative state" (PVS).[39]

DIRECTIVES *

57. A person may forgo extraordinary or disproportionate means of preserving life. Disproportionate means are those that in the patient's judgment do not offer a reasonable hope of benefit or entail an excessive burden, or impose excessive expense on the family or the community.[41]

---

* For the purposes of this volume, we are including only Directives 57 and 58. Directives 55, 56, and 59 through 66 have been omitted.

58. There should be a presumption in favor of providing nutrition and hydration to all patients, including patients who require medically assisted nutrition and hydration, as long as this is of sufficient benefit to outweigh the burdens involved to the patient.

Notes

35. Pope John Paul II, Apostolic Letter, *On the Christian Meaning of Human Suffering (Salvifici Doloris)* (Washington, D.C.: United States Catholic Conference, 1984), nos. 25–27.

36. National Conference of Catholic Bishops, *Order of Christian Funerals* (Collegeville, Minn.: The Liturgical Press, 1989), no. 1.

37. *Declaration on Euthanasia.*

38. Ibid., Part II, p. 4.

39. Committee for Pro-Life Activities, National Conference of Catholic Bishops, *Nutrition and Hydration: Moral and Pastoral Reflections* (Washington, D.C.: United States Catholic Conference, 1992). On the importance of consulting authoritative teaching in the formation of conscience and in taking moral decisions, see *Veritatis Splendor*, nos. 63–64.

41. *Declaration on Euthanasia*, Part IV.

PART FOUR

Ethical and Theological Perspectives

While the preceding sections have discussed the key components of the debate about forgoing or withdrawing artificial nutrition and hydration for persons in a persistent vegetative state and the differing views about them, the present section offers more in-depth theological and ethical analyses of many of these critical and basic assumptions. This cluster of issues, most present from the very beginning of the debate and still unresolved, consists of the following questions

- Is there a moral obligation to preserve human biological life in PVS patients even when there is no hope of recovery of consciousness?
- What counts as burdens and benefits?
- Is the Catholic ethic of forgoing or withdrawing treatment based on the principle of double effect or on the principle of physical and moral impossibility, and what difference does this make?
- May quality-of-life judgments enter into the burden–benefit calculus and, if so, in what sense?
- May life-sustaining treatments be withdrawn only when death is imminent?
- What is the likely intention when withdrawing artificial nutrition and hydration for a patient in PVS?
- Is artificial nutrition and hydration medical treatment or basic care and is the distinction morally relevant?
- Does forgoing artificial nutrition and hydration cause pain and suffering?
- Who should decide about forgoing or withdrawing artificial nutrition and hydration?

The article by Germain Grisez offers arguments against forgoing or withdrawing artificial nutrition and hydration for persons in PVS while those by Thomas Shannon and James Walter, and by Daniel Sulmasy argue for the moral permissibility of such, all claiming that their positions are grounded in and re-flective of the Catholic moral tradition. Each offers persuasive argument but the perspectives and conclusions of the two approaches are substantially different.

Any progress on this issue—that is, achieving some consensus—will require honest and rigorous study of and dialogue on these fundamental questions. Such study and dialogue will likely need to focus on the merits of the positions themselves with regard to each of the fundamental questions, their relationship to the tradition, and their relationship to the current social, technological, and medical context. That is, theological work will need to consider the soundness of the various perspectives on the different questions, whether these perspectives are consistent with the tradition, and whether they are adequate to the current social reality. Thus, critical theological work should precede and inform any intervention by the magisterium. There is much at stake in how these fundamental questions are resolved and not just with regard to forgoing or withdrawing artificial nutrition and hydration. How these questions are addressed will likely impact other forms of life-sustaining treatment as well as our entire ethic and practice of forgoing or withdrawing treatment.

12

The PVS Patient and the Forgoing/ Withdrawing of Medical Nutrition and Hydration

Thomas A. Shannon

James J. Walter

Over the last several decades modern medicine has progressed at a rate that has astonished even its practitioners. Developments in drugs, vaccines, and various technologies have given physicians an incredible amount of success over disease and morbidity as well as allowing them to make dramatic interventions into the body to repair or replace a problematic system or organ. Yet, there are limits we are coming to recognize slowly and only reluctantly. For even many of our best technologies are only halfway technologies, that is, the technology or intervention compensates for a function but cannot cure the underlying pathology or correct the damaged organ. The respirator is probably the most frequently encountered example of this phenomenon.

Another intervention is our capacity to provide nutrition and hydration to those in a persistent vegetative state (PVS). For long-term feeding of such individuals, a gastrostomy tube is inserted directly into the stomach and the liquid protein diet is delivered in a controlled fashion by a pump. If the individual is reasonably healthy and other reflexes are intact, the life expectancy may be several decades.[1] The PVS will not be cured, and the liquid protein serves to maintain the status quo. The question of how to treat these patients medically is now heavily debated nationally and internationally.

In this essay, we will examine the issue in several ways: (1) report on a survey of the U.S. hierarchy on bioethics committees in general and on forgoing or withdrawing nutrition and hydration in particular; (2) propose a structured argument which includes a reconceptualization of "quality of life" judgments; and (3) offer suggestions for the future conduct of this debate.

I. A Survey of the U.S. Hierarchy

General Analysis

In January of 1988 one of the authors (TAS) developed a brief questionnaire which sought information on two broad areas: (1) were there diocesan bioethics committees and, if so, what was their composition, etc., and (2) did dioceses have specific policies on the issue of nutrition and hydration.[2]

One-hundred-sixty-seven questionnaires were sent to the Ordinaries of the U.S. dioceses. Seventy-eight Ordinaries responded. Of these, sixty-two indicated that there was no diocesan bioethics committee, sixteen indicated the existence of such a committee, and of these, seven sent in detailed information, which will be evaluated separately below.

Of those indicating no diocesan committee, eight said that there were committees at local Catholic hospitals. Another eight identified a specific individual within the diocese to whom the Ordinary turned for assistance. Another three indicated the formation of such a committee, either on a diocesan or state level. Finally, one respondent stated there was an inoperative committee.

The survey then asked for a description of the membership of the committee, frequency of meetings, its role, whether there were guidelines, and how it functioned within the diocese. Committee size ranged from nine to twenty-three members, which allowed for a good representation of professions, typically including hospital administrators, physicians, nurses, chaplains, ethicists, lawyers, and other theologians. Six of the committees met monthly, two met bimonthly, and one as needed. Three respondents said their role was to set policy, two were to be advisory, and one was to be primarily educational. Two respondents had no guidelines, and nine indicated some form of guidelines ranging from Church teachings on medical issues to specific pronouncements of the hierarchy over the past decade.

Part 2 of the survey focused specifically on the moral evaluation of feeding tubes. Of the seventy-eight answering, seventeen made no comment on part 2, thirty-seven made some comments, and twenty-two respondents reported no cases of PVS patients in their diocese.

Nine respondents reported knowledge of PVS patients within their dioceses. Of those nine, eight reported figures ranging from one to five per year, and one respondent indicated ten cases in the past year. Eight committees were asked to consider cases and eleven had not been asked. Additionally, four respondents reported that they have specific guidelines they follow in such instances, and eight indicated that they have none.

The survey asked if the committee considered feeding tubes to be a medical technology. Six said yes, four said no, eight gave no answer, and one said "it depends." The respondents were then asked if they considered the use of such feeding tubes to be routine care. Six said yes, four said no, eight gave no answer, and one said "it depends." The next question was whether the removal of a feeding tube from a PVS patient was ordinary or extraordinary care, or if they had no position. Four responded the care was ordinary, four that it was extraordinary, one had no position, nine gave no answer, and nine said "it depends." The final question asked whether removal was an act of involuntary euthanasia, which is direct and forbidden, or indirect and permitted, or no position. Four responded that removal was direct, five that it was indirect, two had no position, four said "it depends," and eight had no answer.

Before turning to an analysis of the seven detailed responses (Documents A-G), we would like to make a few general observations about the data so far.

Given the seriousness of contemporary bioethical questions and their pervasiveness within society, it is surprising so few dioceses have these committees or that so few local Catholic hospitals were indicated as having one. While neither seeking to bureaucratize all life nor to reject appropriate patient and family autonomy, nonetheless such committees on a diocesan or state level serve a useful function, minimally by providing workshops or other resources to hospitals or other groups in the diocese. Of those that are in place, the composition is well represented from a disciplinary perspective, and the committees meet with appropriate regularity. The committees appear to be accessible and, while maintaining patient privacy and confidentiality, there is some degree of openness in the committees.

Part 2 of the questionnaire provides more interesting data. Nine committees had cases brought to them and, taken together, they had a moderately large number of cases—about forty-five. Six committees considered feeding tubes to be a medical technology and also routine care, four thought they were not a medical technology, and one did not consider them routine care. One committee was uncertain in each case. Yet of these committees, only four thought that feeding tubes were ordinary means whose removal constituted active euthanasia.

Four committees considered the technology ordinary, and four judged it to be extraordinary. Four thought their removal to be direct euthanasia while five considered it passive euthanasia. But even more interesting is that nine committees thought that the placing of the technology into the ordinary/extraordinary categories depended on the individual circumstances of the case, and eight thought the same thing about the determination of active or passive euthanasia. This suggests substantial ambiguity about the moral status of feeding technologies for PVS patients.

First, there is a difference over whether the procedure is a medical technology. If a technology, its moral evaluation fits conceptually more easily into the traditional format of ordinary/extraordinary means. If not, one might have to structure the argument differently. Most interesting are the differences in perception between whether the therapy is considered ordinary or extraordinary means, on the one hand, and whether its forgoing/withdrawal is morally evaluated as direct or indirect euthanasia, on the other. This interest is compounded when combined with the additional judgment—on the part of nine and eight respondents respectively—that such a determination "depends" on the circumstances. Such evaluations suggest room for various analyses of the problem and the possible moral acceptability of several resolutions.

Analysis of Specific Guidelines

Seven respondents sent more detailed information about committee make-up and the by-laws governing these committees. We will discuss each document in some detail, but to maintain a promised confidentiality, we will simply refer to these documents as A–G.

Document A suggests that the primary locus for decision making is the local hospital, with the diocesan or proposed state-wide committee serving as a resource. Yet, part of the task of the proposed state-wide committee will be to develop guidelines for the local committee. At present, discussions are ongoing among committees but no consensus has been reached.

Document A affirms a presumption in favor of the use of feeding tubes but states that each case must be examined on its own merits. On the other hand, in very exceptional and extraordinary cases the withdrawal of feeding tubes might be passive and, therefore, permissible euthanasia. Thus, while removal of these tubes is exceptional, their removal is not prohibited either. As the document states it: "each case must be considered on its own merits."

Document B represents the responses from three diocesan hospitals since this diocese has no diocesan committee. B1 indicated that, while there have been cases, the committee did not meet as a committee on them. Rather, individual members of the committee served as resources to the medical staff and the families. This document stated that there is no consensus within the hospital about the issue, and so each case is to be examined on its own merits. The committee understands the practice as passive euthanasia, and thus permissible but also recognizes that there is no consistent position in the hospital.

We detect a problematic area in this document. B1 argues feeding tubes might be withdrawn on the basis

that continued treatment *will result in* prolonged total dependence, persistent pain, or discomfort, or in a *persistent vegetative state*. (Emphasis added.)

However, one wonders how the withdrawal of feeding tubes causes PVS? This technology is used to *support* patients in this condition; its administration does not *result* in PVS.

Document B2 states that their consultation has been on the placement of such technologies rather than on their withdrawal. Since it has no fixed policy, each case must be dealt with individually. Additionally, this committee considers tube feeding to be a medical technology and can become an extraordinary means in specific cases "which must be individually assessed and reassessed." The decisions are to be considered in "light of the effect of this nutrition and/or the burden to the patient which would be experienced." Again, these decisions cannot be based on a broad application of a policy but must be made according to "case specific evaluations."

Document B3 comes from an ethicist at a medical center that has no committee. The respondent indicates that conversations about this problem show that many individuals at the medical center have concerns about the issue. Tube feeding, in this individual's judgment, is a technology, but its moral significance resides in "its function in the ongoing treatment of the patient." Thus, the central issue is: does the treatment contribute to restoring life and health, or does it prolong the patient's dying?

If the former I think it [is] routinely required. If the latter, I judge it foregoable, permissibly not obligatorily foregoable. . . . Tube feeding in some cases is proportionate, hence required, in others, disproportionate, hence not required.

Two other relevant comments were made by this hospital ethicist. First, can feeding tubes ever be withdrawn? If one can

> admit that sometimes tubal feeding need not be *instituted*, then you are already describing conditions which might eventuate *within a case* which justify discontinuing tubal feeding. Put another way, a patient on tubal feeding might become the sort of patient you don't want to begin on tubal feeding. Since you need not start the intervention on the latter patient, why must you stay with it for the former one? (Emphasis in the original.)

Second, never starting or, once begun, removing the tubes is not an intending of death; rather, these decisions indicate that families "recognize and consent to (accept) a dying process which is judged irreversible and imminent."

The two common themes in these three documents from diocesan hospitals are a recognition of the ambiguities in the issue and a strong affirmation of a case-by-case evaluation. The more crucial moral elements are case specific and determining the usefulness of the technology in relation to the condition of the patient. In addition, the suggestion to use the same criteria for not instituting the therapy as the criteria for withdrawing it is a helpful one and could aid in resolving several problems.

Document C is testimony to a state legislature on a natural death act. At issue is the inclusion of a proviso for withholding feeding tubes in a living will. After a strong affirmation of the dignity, sanctity, and value of all human life, this document states:

> The concern to affirm life, however, does not require the maintenance of physiological life by all means. It is recognized that aggressive overtreatment is as ethically unacceptable as is undertreatment. Both lack respect for the dignity and welfare of each person.

This testimony makes four points that lay out several issues very clearly.

1. A clear presumption in favor of life should be established. People who are able to eat, but only with assistance, cannot be discriminated against or be refused appropriate treatment.
2. The law should recognize the right of individuals to be allowed to die in circumstances where medical treatments, including nutrition and hydration, are ineffective or too burdensome for the patient.

3. The law must carefully define useless or ineffective treatment to clearly identify those treatments that offer no benefit of recovery or no relief of pain. The burdens associated with continued medical treatment should be defined in terms of the burdens that an individual experiences in pursuing the goals or ends of life and not defined by a level of invasiveness that may or may not be associated with forced feeding.

4. The clinical setting distinguishes between nutrition and hydration. Although both terms are used as though they are identical, it should be recognized that individuals may not require forced nutrition while still requiring hydration to alleviate thirst, provide comfort, relieve pain, or provide an open channel for IV medications.

Document C is very nuanced and makes careful distinctions. In particular, the document emphasizes the distinction between basic nutrition and hydration that requires time and effort on the part of medical personnel to feed the patient orally and the medical procedures that require total parenteral nutritional support (TPN) or invasive medical techniques to provide nutrition and hydration, e.g., insertion of gastrostomy tubes.

Document D comes from a research center whose writings and contributions were mentioned by many respondents as a source of guidance for their committees. Two major points are made. First, forgoing or withdrawing foods and fluids on the rationale of the "assumption that life itself can be useless or an excessive burden" is morally wrong because it is euthanasia by omission. This carries out the "proposal, adopted by choice, to end someone's life because that life itself is judged by others to be valueless or excessively burdensome." The crucial issues here are the moral intention of those who would withdraw the means of providing nutrition, on the one hand, and the justification for the argument adduced to support such a withdrawal, on the other. For this document, the intention is to end life, and the justification for so acting is that the life is burdensome or useless. This constitutes direct euthanasia.

Second, the forgoing or withdrawing of medically provided nutrition and hydration "do not necessarily carry out a proposal to end life." When certain conditions are met—"if the means employed is [*sic*] judged either useless or excessively burdensome"—one may forgo or withdraw treatment.

Nonetheless, *if it is really useless or excessively burdensome* to provide someone with nutrition and hydration, then these means may rightly be withheld or withdrawn, *provided* that this omission does not carry out a proposal to end the person's life, but rather is chosen to avoid the useless effort or the excessive burden of continuing to provide the food and fluids. (Emphasis in the original.)

Two applications follow. If a person is imminently dying, nutrition may become useless and burdensome, whether administered by tube or otherwise. On the other hand, if the patient is not dying, feeding provides a great benefit: "the preservation of their lives and the prevention of their death through malnutrition and dehydration." Yet even in this instance, this treatment could become useless or futile: "(a) if the person in question is imminently dying, so that any effort to sustain life is futile or (b) the person is no longer able to assimilate the nourishment or fluids thus provided."

On the basis of this analysis, Document D concludes:

We thus conclude that, in the ordinary circumstances of life in our society today, it is not morally right, nor ought it to be legally permissible, to withhold or withdraw nutrition and hydration provided by artificial means to the permanently unconscious or other categories of seriously debilitated but non terminal persons. Food and fluids are universally needed for the preservation of life, and can generally be provided without the burdens and expense of more aggressive means of supporting life.

This document makes a strong argument in favor of such feeding based on the value of human life, the fact that such feeding can provide benefits to the patient and is not generally burdensome, and that the withdrawal of such technology many times includes the intention to end a person's life. Only when the individual is actually dying and/or cannot assimilate nourishment could the feeding be considered an extraordinary means.

Document E represents an advisory opinion of an archdiocese. This opinion bases its position on Pius XII's teaching on ordinary and extraordinary means, the CDF's "Declaration on Euthanasia" and documents from the NCCB Committee for Pro-Life Activities. Document E uses the standards of reasonable hope of success and a determination of excessive burdens as the criteria for decision making. In addition, it recognizes and accepts the presumption of the use of medically providing nutrition and hydration for individuals.

The advisory opinion makes two statements of importance. The first concerns the decision to forgo or withdraw.

It can hardly be denied that in certain circumstances artificial hydration and nutrition can be just as burdensome and useless as other means and under these circumstances would not be obligatory. A Catholic in good conscience can come to the conclusion that in a particular set of circumstances such treatment need not be initiated or continued, because it holds no hope that it will be successful in prolonging life or is unduly burdensome for oneself or another.

The second point concerns the intention involved in ending treatment. Document E argues that "even though the omission may shorten life, the intention is not to bring on death but to spare the patient a very burdensome treatment." These actions could constitute direct euthanasia if the intention is to end the life, but if omitted because they are too burdensome or useless in preserving life, "they do not constitute killing any more than any other such omission."

Document E uses the categories of ordinary and extraordinary means and then draws the conclusions that a decision to forgo or withdraw nutrition can be made in good conscience and that people should not be prevented from doing what is morally permissible. While the document does not encourage forgoing or withdrawal, neither does it prohibit such actions.

Document F supports the removal of nutrition and hydration within the context of the Catholic moral tradition that permits withdrawal of all medical technologies either on the basis that a patient has entered the dying phase or that the technologies are nonbeneficial or burdensome. These evaluations are moral as well as medical: "not what will the treatment do . . . , but will the treatment promote human activities and values."

> Merely maintaining biological life is not evaluated as being in and of itself humanly beneficial. Life is something more than biological existence. Life is a conditional value which couples biological existence with social, spiritual and human activities such as loving, praying, remembering, forgiving and experiencing. Life is all these things.

Consequently, when these activities can no longer be realized, there is no moral obligation to continue medical treatment, unless to relieve suffering. The conclusion that treatment can stop "does not mean that the person is worthless, but that the person has activated all human potential." Thus, there is "no moral requirement to administer artificial nutrition and hydration. In fact it might be violating the person. . . ." Document F concludes on the interesting note that "people feel intuitively that it is wrong and want to find ways to escape imprisonment by technology."

Finally, Document G discusses this issue within the context of policies of life-sustaining treatment. The general context for thinking about this issue is:

> Prolonging physiological function by itself is not of value if it seems all potential for cognitive functions—mental creativity, the capacity to know and to love—if all that is irreversibly destroyed. Respect for life is at the heart of medicine, and a person in such a condition must not be put to death, but may be allowed to die.

The document then considers various forms of supportive care following the decision to allow to die. First, when medical procedures that prolong life are to be withheld or withdrawn, other medical procedures not directed to supportive care may also be omitted. These include lab work, diagnostic procedures, dialysis, nutritional support by mouth or vein, or transfer to an ICU, for example. Measures not to be omitted are: "basic nursing care, including patient hygiene, adequate analgesia, oxygen for comfort, positioning, intake for comfort including intravenous hydration, and nutritional support as tolerated." The document then notes that there may be exceptions to hydration and nutritional support.

> Exceptions to the last two care elements do exist, especially when they offer no benefit or comfort to the patient. Intravenous hydration may not be appropriate when it prolongs or increases discomfort. With careful deliberation, nutritional support may be withheld when all three of the following conditions are present, namely:
>
> [1] The patient has a terminal condition that is irreversible in the final stages.
> [2] The patient is comatose and shows no clinical evidence of experiencing hunger or thirst.
> [3] The patient (or substitute decision-maker) has requested no further treatment.
>
> Other situations not meeting the above criteria for withdrawal or nutritional support care will be decided on a case-by-case basis.

Document G concludes that any treatments during this time of dying should aim at maintaining the dignity of the individual and providing compassion and comfort. The guidelines wisely state that the dying are more in need of comfort and company than treatment and diagnostic procedures.

These documents represent a range of opinions, arguments, and conclusions. All are carefully stated, clearly argued, and located squarely within the Catholic tradition. Yet, different conclusions are drawn from this common heritage, which indicates that the debate is far from finished. There is strong preference for a case by case consideration of the issues and reluctance to have fixed rules to decide cases. On the other hand, there is recognition that some consensus needs to be developed. Finally, there is no enthusiasm or joy about the conclusion that forgoing or withdrawing is morally permissible. While the arguments are sound, the conclusion is reached with sadness and reluctance.

In the second part of this paper we turn to our own contribution to the development of a moral consensus by arguing for the permissibility of forgoing or withdrawing medical procedures that provide nutrition and hydration to PVS patients.

II. An Argument in Support of Forgoing or Withdrawing Medical Nutrition and Hydration

The results of this survey demonstrate to us that the question of forgoing or withdrawing medical procedures for supplying nutrition and hydration is far from settled.[3] In this section we will make our contribution to the debate by proposing arguments supporting the forgoing of this procedure.

The Medical Situation

An important fact about a PVS patient is that he or she is not dying. In these patients the brain stem is intact with the major damage to the brain occurring in the neocortex and cortex. Thus, these patients breathe spontaneously, have their eyes open, have a sleep–wake cycle, their pupils respond to light, and they typically have a normal gag and cough reflex.[4]

With respect to the diagnosis of PVS patients, there is "no set of specific medical criteria with as much clinical detail and certainty as the brain death criteria. Furthermore, even the generally accepted criteria, when properly applied, are not infallible."[5] Furthermore, "It is not uncommon for patients to survive in this condition for five, ten, and twenty years."[6] Survival is contingent on age, economic, familial, and institutional factors, the natural resistance of the body to disease and infection, and changing moral and social views of this condition.

Of critical importance is knowing whether these patients experience pain and/or suffering. Cranford, following the *amicus curiae* brief of the American

Academy of Neurology in the Paul Brophy case, argues that PVS patients "may 'react' to painful and other noxious stimuli, but they do not 'feel' (experience) pain in the sense of conscious discomfort . . ."[7] because the centers of the brain required for these experiences are too compromised to be functional. Thus, PVS patients are not clinically dying, and if they are otherwise in good health and receive appropriate care, they can have a rather long life expectancy. We obviously have the medical capacity to provide nutrition and hydration for these individuals, but the ethical difficulty, of course, is must we do everything we can to sustain their existence in this clinical condition?

The Value of Life

Clearly, the preservation of life is an important goal of the human community in general and of the profession of medicine in particular. Intuitively we know life is valuable and sacred; for were it not, then nothing else would be. Yet, when all is said and done, especially in the Christian framework, life—even human life—is not of ultimate value. Philosophically and politically, we affirm a variety of values that transcend human life: justice, freedom, charity, the good of the neighbor, etc. On the basis of these values or for their sake, we can qualify our protection of individual human lives. Theologically, only God is of ultimate value; all else, no matter how good or valuable, must take second place. Though heresy trials are one, perhaps unfortunate, example of this priority, we also have the celebrated examples of martyrdom and individual self-sacrifice.

This perspective reminds us, particularly in the health care context, that while preserving life is a good—and even a great good—biological life is neither the highest value nor a value that holds ultimate claim on us. To make biological life the ultimate value is to forget our real priorities and to create an idol by making a lesser good our ultimate reality.

The Quality of Life

The meaning and validity of quality of life judgments have been debated in the literature for quite some time.[8] One example in recent decades is Joseph Fletcher's criteria of humanhood.[9] Though his criteria establish standards for being human, they also implicitly argued that life without a certain level of rationality was not human and, consequently, not worth living. Most recently, Robert Jay Lifton's examination of Nazi doctors emphasized the role of the concept of *lebenunvertes Leben*: life unworthy of life.[10] Such unworthiness consisted primarily in being Jewish, but also extended to mental illness and retardation, as well as to severe physical handicaps.[11]

Quality of life judgments can serve as a code for a life judged to be worthless or useless. This orientation comes partially from our consumerist society in which quality is linked with individuals' norms of excellence and is limited only by the horizons of their imagination and desires.[12] This perspective realizes one's worst fears about quality of life judgments because the removal of any transcendent significance or value to human lives gives the state, institutions, or other individuals final control over a person's fate.

The two most crucial levels in the quality of life debate are the evaluative and the normative. At the evaluative level, three points need to be made. First, it is necessary to distinguish clearly and consistently between physical or biological life and personal life (personhood). When this important distinction is not made, quality of life judgments can equivocate between the value of biological life and the value of personhood.[13] This possibility must be removed. Second, physical life is indeed a value that is not conditioned on any property or characteristic of the person. Here, we disagree with Documents F and G which appear to imply such a conditional value of physical life, e.g., its rationality.[14] In our view, physical life is a *bonum onticum*, a true and real value, although created and, therefore, limited. By arguing that physical life as such is a *bonum onticum* and not a conditional value, i.e., a *bonum utile*, we can affirm that all physical lives are of equal *ontic* value and that all persons are of equal *moral* worth. Third, the issue of the evaluative status of physical life may be misplaced from the start. The word "quality" does not and should not refer to a property or attribute *of life*. Rather, the quality that is at issue is the quality *of the relationship* which exists between the medical condition of the patient, on the one hand, and the patient's ability to pursue life's goals and purposes, understood as the values that transcend physical life, on the other.[15] We maintain that this reconceptualization of quality of life judgments is entirely congruent with the substance of the Catholic tradition.

Normatively, those who oppose quality of life judgments fear that life and death decisions will be made solely on the presence or absence of certain qualities or properties that a patient's life possesses. This erodes our duties to protect innocent lives, especially of those most vulnerable in our society.

If one contends that our duties to preserve life are based on a prior judgment of whether a specific quality or property of physical life will result in benefits or good consequences to the patient (personal consequentialism) or to society (social consequentialism), then in our judgment those duties to preserve life are improperly grounded in what the patient earns through social accomplishments or potentialities that the patient's life might possess. We reject such a normative position because it denies, at least implicitly, the equal ontic value of all physical lives.

We argue that one derives the *prima facie* duty to preserve physical life from the ontic value of life and the actual *moral* obligation to preserve life from a teleological, but not consequentialist, assessment of the relationship between the patient's overall condition and his/her ability to pursue life's goals and purposes. The structure of the actual moral obligation is teleological in that the patient's condition is always viewed in relation to the pursuit of life's purposes, and the grounding of the obligation always involves an evaluative assessment of the qualitative relation which exists between these two components. Because physical life is not an absolute value, even those arguing for the sanctity of life position recognize definite limits to the obligation to support life.[16] We should not reject quality of life judgments, but we should rightly reject any normative deriving of our moral duties from the presence of certain properties of physical or personal life.

"Quality of life" judgments, which are judgments strictly circumscribed by an assessment of the benefits and burdens of medical treatment considered in itself and/or of those benefits and burdens that will accrue to the patient as a result of treatment, function appropriately as ways of qualifying our duties to preserve life. Thus, as long as the value of both physical life and personhood is assured at the evaluative and normative levels, we not only support the role of "quality of life" judgments in medicine but also judge them to be indispensable in proper decision making. In our view, then, quality of life judgments properly supplement and enhance the Christian emphasis on the sanctity of life.[17]

The Technological Imperative

We cannot discuss this debate without including a reference to the technological imperative—"if we can do it, we should (or must) do it"—which infers a moral obligation either from a capacity or from the mere existence of a technology.

In the context of high-tech medicine, such an imperative, even if not explicitly subscribed to, is difficult to resist. The same is true even for low-tech or simple technologies. Some medical technologies that administer nutrition and hydration are relatively simple, e.g., parenteral methods of delivering nutrients. Other methods are more invasive, e.g., gastrostomy tubes, and they carry with them potential iatrogenic dangers, such as infection resulting from the surgical creation of the stoma. Yet, they are much less invasive than other procedures and are more risk-free if properly cared for. Furthermore, their use provides a clear and demonstrable benefit: the prolongation of physical life. Indeed, feeding tubes may be unique among all medical technologies in that they almost exceptionlessly deliver on their claims. The technological imperative is augmented by simplicity and predictability of outcome and consequently presents an apparently unassailable case for use. But this very simplicity, ease of use, and ready availability disguises the moral dimension of the technology's use.

One must consider the use with respect to outcome. The outcome, of course, is the preservation of physical life. *Prima facie* such an outcome is valuable, but it must be considered with respect to other values and/or goods, for physical life is not the only or absolute good. Thus, other goods, such as human dignity, ought to be considered. Our point is that, in and of itself, the presence of a technology and the capacity to utilize it constitute at most a *prima facie* case for its use. One cannot automatically or necessarily infer an actual moral obligation from the mere existence or presence of a technology.[18]

The Ordinary/Extraordinary Means Distinction

This well-used distinction can be dated as early as the seventeenth century and has been used by popes and theologians in arguments to determine one's moral obligation to preserve human life.[19] Some maintain that the key element in the traditional use of the distinction is the *classification* of technologies, medicines, or procedures. Consequently, they are considered apart from the patient on whom they are used. Once classified, the moral question is then essentially resolved. In the feeding tube example, the late John Connery, SJ, argued that since nutrition and hydration kept individuals alive, the technology fit the classic definition of ordinary treatment and, therefore, was morally mandatory.[20]

If one shifts the perspective from an abstract classification of technologies to a *patient-centered* approach[21] that gives moral weight to the autonomy of the patient and looks to the impact of these technologies on the patient's medical and nonmedical condition as a whole, one can establish a different moral argument. Here, the expressed wishes of the patient have a legitimate moral claim based on our valuing the dignity of the individual and on our respecting the sacredness of his or her conscience. Second, it is the proportionality or disproportionality of benefits and burdens *to the patient* that makes any medical treatment or procedure, including the medical provision of nutrition and hydration, obligatory or optional. Because the technology can neither ameliorate a PVS patient's general clinical condition nor restore this individual to any state of health where the patient might pursue the values of life, the means are extraordinary and not morally required. Therefore, ordinary and extraordinary are determined not by classifying the technology but by considering its impact on the patient and his/her overall condition. Additionally, and following directly from the above, the distinction must adopt a patient-centered perspective to avoid the technological imperative.

The Burdensomeness of Life

The specific issue here is whether the burdensomeness of the life preserved by the offering of nutrition/hydration can or should be part of the overall assessment of burden in the determination of ordinary/extraordinary as we have just outlined it. Considered only *in itself*, the medical provision of nutrition and hydration would most often be considered ordinary. Thus, for some people any considerations beyond the technology itself would lead to an improper questioning of the value of the patient's life.

We think the concepts of burden and quality of life should be linked. Burden can accrue to the patient precisely through the administration of modern technology and can be a consequence of a life lived merely at the biological level with no hope of restoration or further pursuit of temporal or even eternal goals. In this sense, the burden is iatrogenic. For the PVS patient medicine has reached its limit in bringing this individual to any level of health and wholeness. Again, this patient-centered approach focuses on the conditions under which this valued life is to be lived and seeks to identify what interests of the patient can be achieved. Thus, we argue that burden is to be assessed not only from the perspective of the burdensome effects of the technology itself but, like Document C, also from the perspective "of the burdens that an individual experiences in pursuing the goals or ends of life" as a result of the intervention of the medical technology. Though it is doubtful that the PVS patient would experience this burden personally, the burden is real, even if experienced second-hand by the family and/or by those professionals who must care for the patient.[22]

Fear of Being "Trapped"

The expected benefit of tube feeding is the preservation of life posttrauma or posttreatment so that other important work can go on, e.g., treatment or diagnosis. But there comes a time—sometimes sooner and sometimes later—when one knows that all has been tried and cure is not possible. What was formerly appropriate to do, viz., trying to cure, is now inappropriate, and our efforts must shift to accompanying the patient on his/her final journey.

We agree with Document F that it is precisely here that a family may feel or actually be trapped. Having appropriately initiated medical feeding to preserve life while other tests, procedures, and medications were tried, the family may now be frustrated in its desire to remove the feeding tube. Though such feeding only preserves biological life, attempts to withdraw the feeding may be challenged by medical personnel or by others.

Our fear is that individuals or families may inappropriately refuse to initiate medical procedures for delivering nutrients because of the fear of not being able to withdraw these procedures when that becomes appropriate. Thus, individuals who may genuinely benefit from this type of procedure could be deprived of its goods. Such a situation would be tragic beyond belief. But because of the technological imperative, our near absolutizing of biological life, and the fear of taking personal responsibility in medical decision making, this outcome is almost guaranteed. However, recognizing patient autonomy and shifting to a patient-centered calculation of benefits and burdens in the fashion we have described will counter this unfortunate situation.

Summary

In our judgment, the cumulative effect of our arguments supports the legitimate forgoing or withdrawing of nutrition and hydration to PVS patients. This judgment can properly be reached without supporting any efforts or claims for euthanasia and without making any improper judgments about the worth of a particular life. After carefully considering both the patient's known wishes and the qualitative relation between the patient's medical condition and the pursuit of life's purposes, one may appropriately judge that such a therapy is disproportionate and morally optional. This conclusion seems to be very close to, if not the same as, the judgment contained in Document E.

III. Suggestions for Future Discussion

Having reviewed the results of the survey, the points raised in the various documents submitted to us, and identified several ethical arguments supporting the removal of medical feeding tubes, we wish to make some suggestions for the future conducting of this debate.

Nomenclature

I. THE MISUSE OF "EUTHANASIA" IN THE DEBATE

In our survey Ordinaries were asked whether the diocesan committee considered the removal of feeding tubes from PVS patients to be an act of involuntary euthanasia. The responses are very interesting. Most answered that they considered the withdrawal of these tubes to be "passive or indirect and therefore permitted." A significant number responded that "it depends," and only four respondents answered that this action was "active or direct and therefore forbidden."

The response from the research center, Document D, states that the withdrawal of feeding tubes from PVS patients, except in very limited cases, is an act of "euthanasia by omission," and in most cases anyone who does this has the moral intention to end a life which is considered valueless or excessively burdensome. Two assumptions, frequently cited among those who consider such actions as euthanasia, seem to underlie this conclusion. The first is that the medical provision of nutrients offers a benefit by preserving the life of the patient. The second is that this nourishment should be considered as ordinary *care*, similar to all other types of care.

The moral characterization of the intention of the one authorizing withdrawal as "ending a life" forces this discussion into the context of euthanasia. In its brief to the New Jersey Supreme Court on the Nancy Ellen Jobes' case, the New Jersey Catholic Conference argued that the withdrawal of feeding tubes is "intentional euthanasia."[23] Because we disagree both with the two basic assumptions which underlie this argument and with the description of the moral intention of these acts of withdrawal as killing, we argue that the use of the term euthanasia should be avoided in the debate.

A moral analysis of euthanasia necessarily involves an assessment of the intention. Though they may be motivated by humane reasons, morally, all acts of euthanasia intend the death of the patient, either by commission or by omission, and thus by definition these acts constitute the unjustified killing of a patient. However, we argue that in withdrawing nutrition and hydration the intent is either to end a procedure that no longer benefits the patient or to prevent the person from being entrapped in technology. The patient's death, while foreseen, results from the justified discontinuance of a technology that itself can neither correct the underlying fatal pathology, i.e., the permanent inability to ingest food and fluids orally, nor offer the patient any reasonable hope for what we have defined as quality of life. In our judgment, then, it is inappropriate to characterize the withdrawal of medical nutrition and hydration from PVS patients as euthanasia.

2. THE USE OF "FORGO," NOT "WITHHOLD"

We suggest that in any future discussion of this issue the word "forgo" should be used rather than "withhold." The reason is that "withhold" connotes that something is denied to someone who has some entitlement to it. When family members appropriately decide that a medical treatment will not truly benefit the PVS patient, their decision is to refrain from pursuing what is not useful to the loved one, not to deny something to which the patient has a need or a right. Our intent is twofold: to avoid a begging of the question and to suggest a terminology which allows the argument to come forward and be evaluated on its own merits. The terminology of forgoing and withdrawing, we think, will prevent the argument from becoming confused linguistically and prejudged methodologically.

3. DESCRIPTION OF NUTRITION AND HYDRATION

What to call the nourishment administered to a patient introduces a variety of problems, descriptive as well as symbolic. The terms "food and water" conjure up, among other things, a variety of images depending on taste and ethnic background. They also connote a meal in which one actively participates or, if with others, shares. The symbolism associated with food and water is deep, and rightly so. For they symbolize membership and participation in a community, and to deny these common but significant realities to someone is more than depriving that individual of nourishment; it is cutting him or her off from the community.

The symbolic level of food and water is what inclines several individuals to argue against the removal of nourishment from the PVS patient.[24] The forgoing or the removal of nutrition says that the individual has been marked and put outside the community, outside society. This further signifies the valuelessness of the person and his or her uselessness to the community. Therefore, one must continue to provide this nourishment precisely as a symbol of inclusion.

However, one must also recognize the limits of this symbolism, particularly in the case of PVS patients. First, we have a situation in which the patient is fed and does not eat; the experience is entirely passive. Orderlies or nurses do not deny trays of food to patients nor do they forcibly remove these from the hands of patients. Nutrition and hydration are administered to the patient and the body absorbs them; the feeding process is completely involuntary. Second, the symbolism of the meal is utterly absent, even if others are there. There is no meal, but a medical feeding. Though nourishing, it is difficult to consider such a liquid protein diet as food. For food, in addition to having a certain biological reality, is also a human construct and is more than the sum of its nutritional value. It is the color, texture, aroma, taste and company in which it is shared. For the PVS patient, all of this is absent. To call this nourishment food is to invest it with more meaning than the reality of the situation can bear.

Also, these patients do not consciously experience hunger or thirst. But even if these states were experienced, medical procedures for supplying nutrition and hydration might not relieve the feelings.[25] "Medical nutrition and hydration" seems an appropriate phrase for this form of nourishment because it captures in a nonjudgmental fashion the medical provision of the nourishment as well as the passivity of the experience. The patient is fed and, consequently, the body is nourished, but he or she certainly does not participate in a meal and clearly does not share table fellowship. This terminology also describes the procedure without begging the moral question of whether one ought to provide it, and it avoids the intrusion of inappropriate symbolism. This terminology will keep us from making more of the situation than is there, but it will also keep us from making less of it.

Ordinary and Extraordinary Treatment

I. CHANGE IN THE USE OF THE TERMS

As we noted above, there is a difference in how these traditional terms can be used. For some, the terms are the basis on which the procedure or technology is classified. Once classified, the correct action is relatively clear. If ordinary, the procedure or technology is morally obligatory; if extraordinary, it is morally optional. This schema encounters significant problems when the pace of technological change increases. In addition, the term ordinary in its moral or normative sense has been used to declare a certain technology routine or customary in a medical or descriptive sense. The descriptive use of ordinary generally refers to what is usually done, but this involves little or no moral analysis of what ought to be done.

These equivocations have precipitated a rethinking of the terminology that now aims at the evaluation of the benefit–burden ratio for the patient.[26] Consequently, a procedure is judged ordinary in a normative sense if its effects on the patient provide proportionately more benefits than burdens. Conversely, a treatment is extraordinary in a moral sense if the evaluation produces the contrary conclusion. Thus, these terms are now seen as the *conclusion* of a process of evaluation rather than as a *classification* of a procedure. It is not unusual that a Jehovah's Witness would judge a clinically routine blood transfusion morally extraordinary because of the disproportionate consequences for his or her eternal salvation. Similarly, a person on long term dialysis might conclude in some circumstances that use of this technology is extraordinary because of its impact on diet and life style.

Understanding ordinary and extraordinary as conclusions of an evaluative process rather than as a classification schema permits a much more appropriate use of the terms in the practice of contemporary medicine. Furthermore, the danger of equivocation is now removed, and the meaning of the terms is moral, not descriptive.

2. AUTONOMY

Though the concept of autonomy has undergone some criticism in the last few years because it has been taken to an extreme by functioning independently of or to the exclusion of other values, nonetheless, we might do well to remember the old adage that abuse does not take away its use. Autonomy is an important value, and the proper starting point for these discussions is the expressed wishes of the competent patient. To begin at this point is to respect the dignity of patients and their conscientious decisions. Statements that individuals make about their death or the circumstances of their dying are extremely important. Minimally, they form the foundation of any and all discussions about the initiation or withdrawal of therapy. These statements, which need to be discussed and evaluated in light of the clinical situation and other relevant moral values, always constitute a core element in the final decision about treatment.

3. QUALITY OF LIFE CONSIDERATIONS AND THE GOAL OF MEDICINE

As we have noted, quality of life judgments should not be construed as judgments about the worth of either physical or personal life. They are not concerned with assessing qualities or properties that, when present, make life itself valuable. Rather, these judgments are evaluative and normative claims or assessments about the relation between the patient's overall condition and his or her ability to pursue material, moral and spiritual values that transcend physical life but do not give that life its very meaning and worth. Consequently, quality of life judgments help specify concretely the meaning of the terms "benefits," "burdens," and "best interests" of a patient as well as the limits of medical interventions within a given historical and cultural situation.

Whereas all physical life is of equal ontic worth and all personal life is of equal moral value, the quality of the relation between these lives and the pursuit of values is not equal. Due to multiple factors, some of which have to do with individual genetic endowment and the ways in which we live our lives and some of which are dependent on the nurturing and accessibility of values in a given culture, a large portion of the population is fortunate enough to attain a high quality of life. Other individuals, regrettably, are not as fortunate, and they must live most of their lives pursuing life's purposes at a less than optimal level. But some have no discernible or such a minimal qualitative relation between their overall condition and the pursuit of values that we would argue that those in this last category have no moral obligation to prolong their physical lives. In these cases, all treatment can be withdrawn from them. Not long ago, all PVS patients' lives would have been mercifully ended by their inability to ingest food orally, but the intervention of modern technology today has not been as merciful.

No doubt, one of the principal factors that has provoked this debate has been the ambiguity about the central goal of medicine itself. Medicine rightfully seeks to prevent death, especially an untimely death, to alleviate pain and physical suffering, and to promote health as far as possible. Indeed, these are important goals. However, we argue that all these goals are really subordinate to the more encompassing goal of serving the purposefulness of personal existence.[27] In other words, the central and overarching goal of clinical medicine is to enhance the qualitative relation between the patient's condition and the pursuit of life's goods. Thus, other things being equal, when medicine can intervene to ameliorate the quality of the relation between the patient's condition and the pursuit of life's goals, then such an intervention can be considered a benefit to the patient and is in his or her best interests. On the other hand, because of the overall condition of the patient, when a proposed intervention cannot offer the patient any reasonable hope of pursuing life's purposes at all or can only offer the patient a condition where the pursuit of life's purposes will be filled with profound frustration or with utter neglect of these purposes because of the energy needed merely to sustain physical life, then any medical intervention: (1) can only offer burden to the life treated, (2) is contrary to the best interests of the patient, (3) can cause iatrogenic harm or the risk of such harm, and (4) has reached its limit based on medicine's own principal reason for existence, and thus treatment should not be given except to palliate or to comfort.[28]

Responsibility in Decision Making

I. PLAYING GOD: PEOPLE OR TECHNOLOGY?

When the biotechnological revolution began in earnest and humans discovered new powers and capacities, one of the first slogans to describe this new state of affairs was "playing God." This phrase denoted the power humans now wielded over previously untamed and uncontrolled natural realities. But we detect a shift emerging. Rather than humans playing God, it is now technology that is playing God. Our machines seem to have developed a life and power of their own. How, for example, does someone with an artificial heart die? How does someone on a respirator stop breathing? How does someone with a feeding tube refuse to be nourished? Very often, once in place, there seems to be no way—short of a cosmic power failure—to end the domination of the machine. We are, clearly, much better about removing machines now than we were initially but many are still very reluctant to intervene in the activities of the machinery. Often enough, court intervention is the only recourse the family or guardian has to stop a machine.[29]

Have we surrendered our decision-making powers to machines? Do they "play God" by exercising their untiring, endless vigilance over us and our loved ones? We have not improved our situation much if, indeed, we have turned our appropriate decision making responsibilities over to machines. Although such decisions are dangerous and difficult at times, humans have a legitimate level of responsibility for deciding about the forgoing or withdrawing of treatment. Surrendering that responsibility because a machine is in place is truly the worship of a false god.

2. ROLE OF THE FAMILY

The family typically plays an important role in these decisions because often enough the individual most affected by a decision cannot participate directly. Such involvement is proper because generally the family has a relationship with the patient and knows his or her wishes. The family is normally in the best position to discern the patient's wishes or desires. Thus, they can either relate what the patient actually wanted or, failing that, relate their best judgment of what the patient would have wanted. If the family has no direct knowledge of the patient's wishes, they are still the appropriate decision maker. They have a socially recognized relation to the patient and can be presumed to have the best interests of the patient in mind.

Should conflicts arise that simply cannot be resolved at the local level with the assistance of the physicians, an ethics committee, a patient's rights advocate, the clergy, or other resources, then—and only then in our judgment—is it appropriate to think of turning to the courts for a resolution of the issue. The family, even without knowledge of the patient's wishes, has at least a relation with the patient and is a more appropriate locus for decision making. However, when they cannot resolve the issues and a decision is necessary, then the courts are an appropriate avenue for seeking a decision.

IV. Conclusion

On both practical and theoretical levels, the question of forgoing or withdrawing medical nutrition and hydration from PVS patients appears to have reached no clear consensus inside or outside the Catholic community, although our sense is that many, if not most, people are uncomfortable with continuing this technology when there is no reasonable hope of an improvement in the patient's prognosis. This is not to say that there is an atmosphere of joy about the situation or zeal to begin a withdrawal procedure. Rather, there is a sense of reluctance, a very great sense of caution and care, and a most careful focusing on the moral arguments.

Finally, we wish to highlight two aspects of the debate that we think are particularly crucial. First, the moral intention to forgo or withdraw medical nutrition and hydration is not identical with the intention in euthanasia. This conclusion is confirmed by our own work and in most of the literature. People who advocate the forgoing or the withdrawal of feeding tubes are not advocating any kind of euthanasia policy. The clear intent is to end a procedure that is not proportionately benefiting the person or to release the person from entrapment in technology. Thus, while forgoing or withdrawing feeding tubes is not "medical killing" as some have claimed, it may well be "involuntary medical living." Second, forgoing or withdrawing this technology is argued as a moral option, not as a mandatory practice. Therefore, the conclusion that we share with most authors is either that forgoing or withdrawal is not prohibited or it is within the permitted range of moral activities. We also agree with Document E that individuals who conclude that such a practice is morally appropriate should not be prohibited from acting on that conclusion.

We expect that the debate will continue and that different aspects of it will be further examined. Our hope is that this report and presentation of an argument will help structure that process and assist in its resolution.[30]

Notes

1. The longest case of coma is that of Elaine Esposito, who died 37 years and 111 days after falling into coma. See The President's Commission for the Study of Ethical Problems in Medicine and Biomedical and Behavioral Research, *Deciding to Forego Life-Sustaining Treatment: A Report on the Ethical, Medical, and Legal Issues in Treatment Decisions* (Washington, D.C.: U.S. Government Printing Office, 1983), p. 177, note 16.

2. Some dioceses may not have received a survey either because the See was vacant or because of error on TAS's part. Additionally, not every respondent answered every question. Thus, in terms of data analysis there is no constant "n"; yet, an overall impression can be gained from the data.

3. Throughout the remainder of this essay we have adopted the terminology used by the Hastings Center in describing the technique by which nutrition and hydration are provided to the PVS patient. As defined by the Hastings Center, "medical procedures for supplying nutrition and hydration are medical enteral procedures and parenteral nutritional procedures. . . . Medical enteral procedures are procedures in which nutritional formulas and water are introduced into the patient's stomach or intestine by means of a tube, such as a gastrostomy tube or nasogastric tube. . . . Parenteral nutritional procedures are procedures in which nutritional formulas and water are introduced into the patient's body by means other than the gastrointestinal tract. Such procedures include total parenteral nutritional support (TPN), in which a formula capable of maintaining the patient for prolonged periods is infused into a vein—usually a large, central vein in the patient's chest—and intravenous procedures in which water and/or a formula supplying limited nutritional support is introduced into a peripheral vein." The Hastings Center, *Guidelines on the Termination of Life-Sustaining Treatment and the Care of the Dying* (Briarcliff Manor, N.Y.: The Hastings Center, 1987), pp. 140–41.

4. For a more detailed discussion of the condition of a patient in persistent vegetative state, see Ronald E. Cranford, "The Persistent Vegetative State: The Medical Reality (Getting the Facts

Straight)," *Hastings Center Report* 18 (February/March, 1988): 27–32. Also, see The President's Report, *Deciding to Forego Life-Sustaining Treatment*, pp. 174–81.

5. Cranford, "The Persistent Vegetative State," p. 29.

6. *Ibid.*, p. 31

7. *Ibid.* In addition, see the recent "Position of the American Academy of Neurology on Certain Aspects of the Care and Management of the Persistent Vegetative State Patient," reprinted in *Medical Ethics Advisor* 4 (August, 1988): 111-13.

8. For example, see George J. Annas, "Quality of Life in the Courts: Earle Spring in Fantasyland," *The Hastings Center Report* 10 (August, 1980): 9–10; Daniel Callahan, *Setting Limits* (New York: Simon & Schuster, 1988), pp. 187–93; John R. Connery, SJ, "Quality of Life," *Linacre Quarterly* 53 (February, 1986): 26–33; Brian V. Johnstone, CSSR, "The Sanctity of Life, the Quality of Life and the New 'Baby Doe' Law," *Linacre Quarterly* 52 (August, 1985): 258–70; Edward W. Keyserlingk, *Sanctity of Life or Quality of Life in the Context of Ethics, Medicine and Law* [A study written for The Law Reform Commission of Canada] (Ottawa: Minister of Supply and Services Canada, 1979), pp. 49–72, 75–105, and 185–90; Richard A. McCormick, SJ, "A Proposal for 'Quality of Life' Criteria for Sustaining Life," *Hospital Progress* 59 (1975): 76–79; *idem*, "The Quality of Life, The Sanctity of Life," *Hastings Center Report* 8 (February, 1978): 30–36; Warren T. Reich, "Quality of Life," in *Encyclopedia of Bioethics*, Vol. 2, ed. Warren T. Reich (New York: The Free Press, 1978), pp. 829–40; and Warren T. Reich, "Quality of Life and Defective Newborn Children: An Ethical Analysis," in *Decision Making and the Defective Newborn: Proceedings of a Conference on Spina Bifida and Ethics*, ed. Chester A. Swinyard (Springfield, IL: Charles C. Thomas, 1978), pp. 489–511.

9. Joseph Fletcher, "Indicators of Humanhood: A Tentative Profile of Man," *Hastings Center Report* 2 (November, 1972): 1–4.

10. Robert Jay Lifton, *The Nazi Doctors: Medical Killing and the Psychology of Genocide* (New York: Basic Books, 1986), p. 21.

11. For an interesting contrast between the Nazi interpretation of "quality of life" and what contemporary authors tend to mean by this criterion, see Cynthia B. Cohen, "'Quality of life' and the Analogy with the Nazis," *The Journal of Medicine and Philosophy* 8 (1983): 113–35.

12. Albert R. Jonsen, "Purposefulness in Human Life," *The Western Journal of Medicine* 125 (July, 1976): 5.

13. For example, Warren Reich's theological position grounds both the value and the equality of "human life" in the belief that "all men are created as persons in the image of God" (Reich, "Quality of Life and Defective Newborn Children," p. 504). His use of the phrase "human life" is ambiguous here and therefore misleading. The context of his argument is a critique of what he believes to be Richard A. McCormick's position on the value of *physical life*, yet Reich completes his argument by referring to *persons* and their nature and value as images of God.

14. In fact, several contemporary Catholics have given the impression that the value of physical life is dependent on some inherent property or attribute that, when present, gives physical life its value. It is possible that this way of phrasing the value of physical life is due to the lack of a terminology in the contemporary discussion that can mediate between the two traditional categories of value, viz., *bonum honestum* and *bonum utile*. For example, see Kevin D. O'Rourke, OP, and Dennis Brodeur, *Medical Ethics: Common Ground for Understanding* (St. Louis, MO: The Catholic Health Association of the U.S., 1986), p. 213; Richard A. McCormick, *How Brave A New World?*:

Dilemmas in Bioethics (Washington, D.C.: Georgetown University Press, 1981), pp. 405–7; and David Thomasma *et al.,* "Continuance of Nutritional Care in the Terminally Ill Patient," *Critical Care Clinics* 2 (January, 1986): 66.

15. See James J. Walter, "The Meaning and Validity of Quality of Life Judgments in Contemporary Roman Catholic Medical Ethics," *Louvain Studies* 13 (Fall, 1988): 195–208, esp. p. 201.

16. For example, see John R. Connery, SJ, "Prolonging Life: The Duty and Its Limits," *Linacre Quarterly* 47 (May, 1980): 151–65; Johnstone, "The Sanctity of Life, The Quality of Life," esp. pp. 265–69; and Reich, "Quality of Life and Defective Newborn Children," esp. pp. 505–9.

17. Keyserlingk also argues a similar position in his report for the Law Reform Commission of Canada. See his *Sanctity of Life or Quality of Life,* esp. pp. 49–72.

18. We agree with the report from the Hastings Center that "All invasive procedures for supplying nutrition and hydration—all enteral and parenteral techniques—should be considered procedures that require the patient's or surrogate's consent. . . ." The Hastings Center, *Guidelines on the Termination of Life-Sustaining Treatment and the Care of the Dying,* p. 61.

19. See, Gerald Kelly, SJ, *Medico-Moral Problems* (St. Louis, MO: The Catholic Hospital Association, 1958), pp. 128–41.

20. John R. Connery, SJ, "The Clarence Herbert Case: Was Withdrawal of Treatment Justified?" *Hospital Progress* 65 (February, 1984): 32–35 and 70.

21. Recently, several authors have argued for a patient-centered approach in clinical decision making. For example, see Robert M. Veatch, *Death, Dying, and the Biological Revolution: Our Last Quest for Responsibility* (New Haven: Yale University Press, 1976); and James J. Walter, "Food & Water: An Ethical Burden," *Commonweal* 113 (November 21, 1986): 616–19.

22. Though we have refrained from making any judgment about the financial burden either on society or on insurance companies in providing funds for PVS patients, the fact that there are approximately ten thousand of these patients in the U.S. strongly inclines us to agree with Daniel Callahan that "It is hard to see how a debate on that reimbursement issue can be forestalled much longer." See Callahan's "Vital Distinctions, Mortal Questions: Debating Euthanasia & Health-Care Costs," *Commonweal* 115 (July 15, 1988): 404. It is important to note here that the *Declaration on Euthanasia* and Document E, both following Pius XII, do permit one to assess the burden on the family or on the community in judging whether a treatment is disproportionate. See the *Declaration on Euthanasia* in *Origins* 10 (August 10, 1980): 16.

23. New Jersey State Catholic Conference Brief, "Providing Food and Fluids to Severely Brain Damaged Patients," in *Origins* 16 (January 22, 1987): 583. The Conference was following the Lutheran theologian Gilbert Meilaender in his "On Removing Food and Water: Against the Stream," *Hastings Center Report* 14 (December, 1984): 11–13. An opposing position was taken by Bishop Gelineau of Providence, Rhode Island, in the Marcia Gray court case. See his statement in *Origins* 17 (January 21, 1988): 546–57.

24. For example, see Daniel Callahan, "On Feeding the Dying," *The Hastings Center Report* 13 (October, 1983): 22.

25. The Hastings Center, *Guidelines on the Termination of Life-Sustaining Treatment and the Care of the Dying,* p. 59.

26. See the *Declaration on Euthanasia* where the terminology has shifted to a discussion of proportionality between the benefits and the burdens.

27. Jonsen, "Purposefulness in Human Life," p. 6.

28. Walter, "The Meaning and Validity of Quality of Life Judgments," p. 207.

29. There have been several court cases recently involving patients in a persistent vegetative state. Two of the more notable cases are Paul Brophy and Nancy Ellen Jobes.

30. Support for the survey was provided by the Research Development Council of Worcester Polytechnic Institute, and the authors acknowledge their gratitude for this assistance.

13

Should Nutrition and Hydration Be Provided to Permanently Unconscious and Other Mentally Disabled Persons?

Germain Grisez

The title of this article can be understood either as a legal or as an ethical question. I treat it here only insofar as it is an ethical question—that is, a moral issue.[1] But I hope my treatment will contribute to the current debate about what law ought to require in this matter. For, of course, questions about what law *should* require are, at least in large part, moral questions.

In its reflection on moral questions, ethics has a task very different from that of legal studies which focus on the making and application of social rules. For ethics tries to *discover* what is good and right for persons and groups of persons, considered insofar as they are agents. In other words, ethics tries to learn the truth about what ways of acting will make persons and communities truly flourish. Thus, my aim in writing this article is not to try to use ideas and words to channel anyone's behavior, but to articulate my own effort to arrive at a sound view on the question, in the hope that doing so will help others who want to know what they ought to do about it.

I did not formulate the title of this article, but accepted it as a question put to me. I take "permanently comatose" to refer to all who are in fact permanently unconscious, no matter what their specific condition or its underlying cause.[2] I presuppose here that even comatose human individuals are persons.[3]

For brevity's sake, I shall use the single word "comatose" to refer to the permanently unconscious, and the single word "food" to refer to nutrition and hydration.

171

For the purpose of this article, I set aside two types of cases:

First, sometimes a choice is made to kill someone, and that choice is carried out by withholding food. (It seems to me that this is exactly what has been done in some of the widely publicized cases.) Now, if food is withheld precisely in *order to* kill someone, that calculated omission, I believe, is homicide and cannot be morally justified. I have argued for this view elsewhere and shall take it for granted here.[4]

Second, sometimes a comatose or other mentally disabled person is dying, and providing food will not prolong life or give the person comfort, and perhaps even will increase discomfort. I agree with what seems to be a general consensus that in such cases food should not be provided. For, just as is true of any other sort of care or treatment, the reason for providing food is to benefit the person being cared for, and therefore, when doing so is no benefit, and perhaps is a burden, it is not reasonable to continue trying to provide food.

Thus, this article concerns only cases of the following sort: no choice is made to kill the comatose or otherwise mentally disabled person, the person is not dying, but the burdens of care and its limited benefits make some or all of those concerned wonder whether it is right to continue providing food.

I also set aside the method of feeding called "total parenteral feeding" or "hyperalimentation."[5] It differs significantly in its burdens from other methods of feeding and is used in few if any cases to sustain comatose persons. So, I do not consider it relevant to the general question to be treated here.

In 1986 I published a lecture in which I dealt with the part of the issue bearing on *comatose* persons. In that lecture, I said:

> If a patient is not in imminent danger of death but is in an irreversible coma, as the late Miss Karen Quinlan was, life-support care more sophisticated than ordinary nursing care is very costly. It seems to me that such costly care exceeds a permanently comatose person's fair share of available facilities and services. Thus, I believe that when Miss Quinlan was removed from intensive care, she ought not to have been placed in a special care facility, but should instead have been sent home or cared for in the hospital with only the sorts of equipment and services available in an ordinary household. These do not include feeding by tube, and Miss Quinlan could not be fed otherwise. Thus, if I am right, she should not have been fed. Not feeding patients in irreversible coma would cause their early death, and it would be wrong to omit feeding them to hasten their death. But a proxy could decide against care in a special nursing facility out of fairness to others, and accept the patient's death as a side effect.

Does it follow that no one is entitled to a lifetime of care, including feeding by tube, at the level Miss Quinlan received? No, because the same principle of fairness by which the cost of that level of care is excessive for people in irreversible coma will require as much or more care for many other patients. This can be seen by applying the Golden Rule, which expresses what fairness demands, to various cases. We all know that each of us might sometime be in irreversible coma, might sometime need public funding of long-term treatment for some other condition, and must always pay taxes. I think we can honestly say that we are willing to limit treatment of ourselves and those we love, if ever in irreversible coma, to ordinary nursing care, without feeding by tube. By setting this limit, we will keep publicly funded special care facilities free for other patients, and avoid increasing taxes to provide additional facilities of this sort. But if we or someone we loved were conscious and able to do some good things and have some good experiences, we would want a lifetime of care at or even above the level Miss Quinlan received, including feeding by tube, if necessary, and we would want public funds to be available for what was needed. Hence, we cannot fairly limit others' care if they are in this condition. Nor can we reject the taxation required to provide facilities for such people.[6]

I continued to hold this view until quite recently, and so thought that it is not reasonable to provide food to *comatose* persons. However, I now think that in our society food should be provided, as a rule, even to such persons. Six considerations led me to change my mind on this matter. I shall first list them briefly, and then articulate in the form of an argument the view to which they have led me.

List of Considerations

First, I had assumed that the class of comatose persons is well defined and that members of the class usually can be picked out easily and with certainty. But I noticed the conflicting testimony of different experts in some of the widely publicized cases, and I discussed the problem with specialists in neurology. As a consequence, it now seems to me that "comatose" refers not to a clear-cut type of case but to a spectrum of cases in which damage to the nervous system has resulted from various causes, damage varies considerably in degree, and serious difficulties can arise in the attempt to make a diagnosis.

Second, I had assumed that feeding a comatose person by tube is in itself complicated and difficult, so that such a person could be cared for only in a special care facility. But I talked with nurses experienced in home health care, and learned that this is not so. Some families care for a comatose family member at home.

Third, I had assumed that feeding a comatose person by tube is in itself expensive. But I was not paying attention to the distinction between the cost of feeding such a person and the total cost of caring for him or her. Most of the cost is for other elements of care: providing a room with suitable furnishings and equipment, keeping it warm, having someone present to do *everything* that must be done (not only to provide food), and so forth. The food itself costs very little, and those who care for comatose persons spend only a small part of their time in feeding them.

Fourth, I had assumed that once a person is comatose, the only human good at stake is his or her life. But, in talking with people about family experiences in caring for debilitated members, I realized that a decent family has another personalistic reason to care for its members and never to abandon any of them except in the most extreme circumstances—for instance, when the family must abandon one member to save the rest. People find it hard to articulate this personalistic reason, but it amounts to something like this: Caring for people—especially providing food and other elemental forms of care—affirms their dignity as persons, expresses benevolence toward them, and maintains the bond of human communion with them. Therefore, if, as I have always believed, even a comatose human individual is a person, feeding that person also serves this personalistic good, which I shall refer to as the good of *human solidarity*.

I had assumed that tube feeding is used only to sustain persons who cannot ingest food in the normal way. But in talking with physicians and nurses who are directly acquainted with current practices in institutions where the severely retarded and very senile are maintained, I learned that uncooperative persons sometimes are fed by tube simply because pouring a formula down a tube is easier, faster, and thus cheaper than patiently feeding such people in the way that parents feed uncooperative babies. Learning this, I realized I had overlooked the fact that the criterion which I had suggested—namely, being conscious and able to do some good things and have some good experiences—excludes not only the comatose but many people who, although conscious, are mentally disabled to such an extent that they never have been (or, at least, never again will be) able to do any good thing or have any good experience.

Sixth, I had assumed that not caring for the comatose would make special care facilities available for other persons without increasing taxes. But the more I learn about the economics of the health-care system, the more I am inclined to think that savings at one point are likely to be lost to the always increasing costs of health care rather than to be put to better use at some other point. So, I am now far less optimistic about the likely economic consequences of withholding or withdrawing care from the comatose.

In view of these considerations, I now believe that in our affluent society and others like it, food ordinarily should be provided even for comatose persons and *a fortiori* for other mentally disabled persons. But the limits of this position should be noticed. It leaves two kinds of cases in which it would be right to withhold or withdraw food from the comatose, and perhaps from some other people.

First, in a community that, unlike our affluent society, is so poor that caring for the comatose and other disabled persons would deprive still others, such as healthy children, of necessities, I think it would be reasonable to use the limited available resources to feed and care for those likely to receive greater benefits from the use of those resources.

Second, I do not think that fairness always requires what it ordinarily requires, for fairness does not require us to feed someone now comatose who when formerly competent envisaged the future situation, and clearly and freely rejected food in that situation, should it ever come about.

In mentioning someone's rejection of food, I am not referring to offhand remarks made once upon a time by any and every person who is now comatose. What I have in mind, rather, are the decisions of people who were competent enough that they could have made a valid will, and who carefully considered the possibility of a future situation in which they would be certifiably comatose. And by "rejection of food" I mean that they made it perfectly clear that, should they ever be in the condition which they envisaged, they wanted to forego care, including food, in order, for instance, to save others the cost of caring for them. It seems to me that such people are not trying to commit suicide and that they have the moral right to concede their own claim upon others for care.

Of course, it does not follow that anyone is entitled to make such a concession on behalf of someone else. For while one often may set aside one's own rights in a spirit of self-sacrifice, one never may set aside the rights of others.

Within its limits, I think that the position I now hold concerning feeding the comatose and other mentally disabled persons is in the line with the Golden Rule. For the Golden Rule requires us to feed even the comatose if we would reasonably want others to feed us or those we hold near and dear if we or our loved ones were ever comatose. And if, as I shall now try to show, providing food to the comatose significantly benefits them and others concerned without still more significantly burdening either the comatose themselves or others concerned, then we *could reasonably* want others to feed us and those we love, even if we or they were in a comatose condition.

First I shall discuss the burdens of feeding the comatose, then its benefits.

Burdens of any sort of care or treatment are those negative aspects of it which can be good reasons for foregoing, withholding, or withdrawing it. Among such negative aspects are organic side effects, cost, painfulness, psychological repugnance, and interference with worthwhile outward behavior or inner activities.[7]

Persons who envisage a future situation in which they would be comatose might reasonably decide to forego care should that situation arise because of its cost and, perhaps, because of psychological repugnance toward being fed by tube. But these aspects of care are not burdens for persons who did not earlier forego care and who have now become comatose. These comatose persons neither bear the costs of their own care nor, presumably, *experience* any of its negative aspects. For if they do experience any burdens of the care they are receiving, they cannot be called "comatose" and also might experience the pain of dying from hunger and thirst.

Of course, persons can suffer burdens which they do not experience. But what burdens can a comatose person suffer? Indignities, certainly, that is, violations implying denial of their status as persons—for example, a comatose person could be used as a sex object or dumped into the garbage. But caring for comatose persons, including feeding them by tube, does not in itself constitute an indignity. (Rather, to say that being fed by tube is an indignity is merely to express an observer's feeling of repugnance.) Moreover, I fail to see that feeding the comatose imposes any other burden on them personally.

What about burdens to others? Admittedly, others must bear the cost of feeding the comatose. But many will argue that a far more important burden is that experienced by a comatose person's loved ones, whose joy in living and peace of mind are damaged or even destroyed by having someone they care about maintained in a hopeless condition with no resolution of the situation in sight.

This argument is emotionally moving but fallacious. Plainly, being comatose is a miserable state, and neither option—to maintain people in that state or to stop maintaining them—is attractive. The situation is similar in this respect to many others that are inescapable in the human condition: nothing one can do *feels* "right." So, as a comatose person's loved ones watch what is done to provide food and other care, they experience a negative aspect in the situation—in other words, they experience a great and undeniably real burden. But it is not a burden of the comatose person's feeding or other care. Rather, it is the burden of that person's extreme disability. Of course, this burden will be eliminated if food is withheld, but only because the comatose person will be eliminated. Thus, to decide not to feed a comatose person in order to end the burden that his or her loved ones experience is to choose to kill that person in order to end the miserable state in which he or she now lives. And that choice is homicidal.

As I narrated above, when I began to pay attention to the distinction between the cost of feeding the comatose and the total cost of caring for them, I realized that by itself the cost of feeding them—which does constitute a burden on others—is comparatively insignificant. For example, providing the bed and services for Miss Quinlan to live out her days cost the public a good deal, but her formula and the work of feeding it to her made up only a small part of the total cost of caring for her. Yet those who oppose providing food for the comatose on the ground of cost invariably seem to have in mind, as I formerly did, the total cost of caring for such persons, not the small cost of feeding them.

This fact leads to a dilemma for anyone who uses cost to justify a decision not to feed a comatose person. Either food is withheld precisely as a means of saving the total cost of care or, at least, food is withheld as part of a more inclusive decision to save that total cost. If food is withheld precisely as a means of saving the total cost of care, the choice is to kill the comatose person, since the means achieves its end only by starving the person to death and rendering unnecessary any further care (except for disposal of the corpse). But, as I said near the beginning of this article, the choice to kill the person would be homicidal and, therefore, morally unjustifiable. If, however, food is withheld as part of a more inclusive decision to save the total cost of care, the issue no longer is whether comatose persons should be fed or not, but whether they should be cared for or abandoned. But the choice to abandon comatose persons bears on every element of their care, and so it cannot be justified by considerations which concern only either the technique by which they are fed or the appropriateness of medical treatment for persons in their situation. So, the real but hidden issue emerges: in our affluent society, can we justify abandoning the comatose in order to save the cost of caring for them as we care for others who cannot care for themselves?

Although the issue thus shifts, it remains necessary to discuss the benefits of caring for comatose persons. For some will hold that even if the comatose remain persons, caring for them neither benefits them nor anyone else. Against that view, it seems to me that caring for the comatose and other less severely mentally disabled persons carries with it two important benefits: it keeps them alive and it maintains human solidarity with them.

Many Deny Benefits

Many deny that keeping people alive benefits them when there is no prospect that they will ever gain or regain the use of their specifically human capacities. For example, Kevin O'Rourke, OP, focusing on the tube feeding of comatose persons, argues that it is useless to sustain life unless doing so helps a person to pursue "the purpose of life," and writes: "In order to pursue the purpose of life, one needs some degree of cognitive-affective function."[8] Richard A. McCormick, SJ, makes a more general assertion along similar lines: "Life is a value to be preserved precisely as providing the condition for other values and therefore insofar as these other values remain attainable. To say anything else is, I submit, to make an idol of mere physical existence."[9]

In denying that "mere physical existence" is inherently good, O'Rourke, McCormick, and all who share their views presuppose that a person's life has only the status of an instrumental good—something which human persons have and use for their specifically human purposes, but, nevertheless, something which remains really distinct from what human persons are. For if O'Rourke and McCormick did not presuppose that human life is only an instrumental good, they could not hold that it is pointless to preserve a person's life unless "some degree of cognitive-affective function" can be restored or "other values remain attainable." But a person's life is not merely an instrumental good. For it is the very actuality of his or her living body, and—although human persons also have spiritual powers and acts which cannot be reduced to bodily capacities and functions—a human being's living body is the bodily person. To deny this is to accept a position which requires some sort of dualistic theory of human persons—that is, a theory according to which human beings are inherently disembodied realities who only have, inhabit, and use their bodies.[10]

No form of dualism is rationally defensible. For every dualism sets out to be a theory of one's personal identity as a unitary and subsisting self—a self always organically living but only discontinuously conscious and now and then inquiring, choice-making, and using means to achieve purposes. But every form of dualism renders inexplicable the unity in complexity that we experience in every act we consciously do. For instance, as I write this, I am the unitary subject of my fingers hitting the keys, the sensations I feel in them, the thought I am expressing, my commitment to write this article, and my use of the computer to express myself. So, *within the one reality that I am*, consciousness and bodily behavior coexist, and dualism starts out to explain me. But every dualism ends by denying that there is any *one* something of which to be the theory. It does not explain me; it tells me about two things, one a nonbodily person and the other a nonpersonal body, neither of which I can recognize as myself.[11]

It follows that, whatever persons are, they cannot be essentially disembodied realities. So, a human person includes a body; one's living body is an intrinsic part of one's personal reality; one does not merely possess, inhabit, and use one's body as an instrument. And so, human life, which is the very actuality of a person's body, is a good intrinsic to the person, not a merely instrumental good for the person. Therefore, contrary to what O'Rourke, McCormick, and others think, human life is inherently good, and so it does not cease to be good when one no longer can enjoy a degree of cognitive-affective function or attain other values.

There are two further implications—that are often overlooked or unmentioned by its proponents—of the thesis that human life is merely an instrumental good to be sustained only so long as it is an effective condition for attaining other goods inherent in human persons.

First, if life is not a good inherent in persons, then the choice to kill a person is wrong, not in itself, but only insofar as it undermines other goods which are inherent in persons. In other words, since O'Rourke, McCormick, and others who share their view see no benefit whatsoever to certain persons in keeping them alive, they would, if they were consistent, see no harm to those same persons in killing them. But that view clearly would be contrary to the Judeo-Christian tradition.

Second, if life were worth sustaining only for those who could attain further goods, then the lives of many permanently and severely mentally disabled people would hardly be more worth sustaining than the lives of the comatose. For many such disabled persons are no more able than the comatose—according to my own earlier formulation—"to do some good things and have some good experiences." Hence, the denial that human life is a good inherent in persons logically points to killing not only the comatose but many conscious people who live, often quite wretchedly, in public institutions or private nursing homes.

Some May Suspect "Slippery Slope" Argument

At this point, some will think that I have made a so-called slippery-slope argument, and they may suppose that it vitiates the whole argument I am trying to articulate in this article. The latter supposition certainly would be false: the main line of my argument is complete in itself and does not require this and the three previous paragraphs. What is more, this incidental argument of mine differs from a slippery-slope argument. For my argument brings out *logical* implications of the assumption that human life is only an instrumental good while a slippery-slope argument would point to the psychosocial dynamics that do not logically imply but which in fact might lead from killing the comatose to killing other mentally disabled persons.

Does it follow from my argument against the view shared by O'Rourke and McCormick that one must "make an idol of mere physical existence" and treat human life as an "absolute good" that must be preserved at all costs, regardless of the burdens of doing so and the benefits which might be gained by using available means to pursue other human goods? Not at all. But two things do follow from the fact that life is a good intrinsic to the person. First, any choice to kill a person is a choice contrary to his or her good, and so is a choice inconsistent with rational love (though, perhaps, consistent with a feeling of affection) toward that person. Thus, one cannot love any neighbor, even a comatose person, and at the same time choose to kill that person. Second, acts which effect nothing more than keeping a person alive, no matter what that person's condition, do really benefit the person, even if only in a small way, and so, if not done for some ulterior reason, do express love toward the person.

This brings us to the second benefit of caring for comatose persons rather than abandoning them: caring for them maintains human solidarity with them— that is, it affirms their dignity as persons, expresses benevolence toward them, and maintains the bond of human communion with them. This personalistic good is realized both in those who receive care and in those who provide it.

Some will deny that maintaining human solidarity with a comatose person in any way benefits him or her, for they will deny that this or any other personalistic good can be realized in a person who is permanently unconscious. However, as I noted above, permanently unconscious people plainly can be burdened insofar as they can suffer indignities; by the same token, such persons can be benefited by being cared for out of a love which respects their dignity. Moreover, one can maintain the bond of human communion with permanently unconscious persons, even though they cannot enjoy the good experiences normally characteristic of this bond as it exists among conscious persons. For this bond is a moral reality, which is maintained essentially by fidelity of will and action. For example, a husband who is faithful to his comatose wife maintains marital communion with her, and so truly benefits not only himself (by continuing to be a good husband) but her, although she cannot consciously enjoy this benefit. Similarly and generally, families and larger communities that faithfully care for their comatose members maintain human communion with them and thereby benefit not only themselves (by continuing to be loving families and genuine communities) but also their comatose members.

Some, of course, will reply that a husband who is faithful to his comatose wife is a sentimental fool whose perseverance is pointless because it benefits nobody, and whose refusal to adjust to the realities of his situation only prevents him from getting on with his life. The questions such a reply opens up are so profound that, within the limits of this article, I can only sketch them out. Underlying the reply, it seems to me, are modern conceptions of the human person, of human community, and even of morality itself that are very different from those of the Judeo-Christian tradition. According to that tradition, human individuals become good persons and form community by loving one another, and they effectively love one another by freely making and faithfully fulfilling self-determining commitments to use their gifts and resources in the service of meeting common needs and pursuing common ideals. According to the modern view that underlies the denial of the worth of a husband's fidelity to his comatose wife, human individuals become good persons by working to satisfy their desires as a whole and in the long run; they form community inasmuch as those desires include some that are based on sympathy and others that arise from the inescapable dependence of human beings on one another; and practical choices are either rationally determined by these goals and the means available for pursuing them or are foolish—that is, uninformed by the realities, short sighted, and emotionally motivated. Because the Judeo-Christian tradition locates human goodness in the free and mutual self-gift that transcends every given desire, it presupposes and affirms freedom of choice. Because the modern view locates human goodness in the rational satisfaction of given desires, it has no need for freedom of choice and leads to its denial (although the modern view exalts the liberty of individuals and groups to use available means in the rational pursuit of the goals that will satisfy their desires). Although the argument is a long one, I think it can be shown philosophically, without assuming premises from religion or morality, that human persons can make free choices and, from this, that the modern view of human goodness oversimplifies human possibilities and so provides a foreshortened, distorted view of what human life is all about.[12]

Comparing Burdens and Benefits

Having considered both the burdens and the benefits of caring for comatose persons, I now compare the two. The only real burden is the cost; the benefits are both in keeping these persons alive and in maintaining human solidarity with them. The latter good is, I believe, at the heart of the moral truth about this question. If we understand human solidarity and the precise way in which it is at stake in the question of caring for comatose persons, we shall see both why in general we should care for them and why under certain conditions we need not care for them.

Competent persons who envisage the future situation of being comatose, and who clearly and freely reject food in that situation, should it ever come about, need not he choosing to kill themselves. They can, instead, be choosing, both to avoid being kept alive *by a method* toward which they feel psychological repugnance and to free others of the burden of the cost of caring for them. If people who have made and adequately communicated such a decision become comatose, others can comply with their choice without in any way violating human solidarity with them. For under these conditions, not caring for the comatose person is not abandonment. Rather, by respecting the comatose person's wishes, others express their benevolence, affirm that person's dignity, and maintain the bond of human communion with him or her.

Again, other grave obligations could take priority over the duty to care for the comatose or other mentally disabled members of a family or larger community. When other obligations do take priority, withholding care does not have the significance of elective abandonment, namely, the breaking off of human solidarity. That is why an impoverished society need not deprive other members of necessities to care for the comatose. But in our affluent society, to abandon

comatose persons who never clearly communicated to others a personal decision to forego care would be to break off human communion with them and
to deny their personhood. Abandoning them would be tantamount to dumping
them into the garbage.

This conclusion can be defended by answering some arguments and objections from the opposing point of view.

Many who oppose feeding the comatose argue that artificial feeding is a
form of medical treatment, and so must be evaluated precisely as therapy. As
such, they claim, it is useless treatment, for the comatose, by definition, cannot be restored to health. Others have answered this argument by pointing out
both that even artificial feeding is an elemental form of care, which has great
human significance, and that medical treatment that preserves whatever remains
of human life and functioning is not entirely pointless even if it is impossible
to restore health.[13]

I think the main thrust of these answers is sound, but they err both insofar
as they focus on feeding the comatose and insofar as they see the significance of
feeding as merely expressive or symbolic. So, it seems to me, the answer to the
argument that feeding the comatose is a form of medical treatment is clarified
and strengthened by two of the points I made earlier: that the real issue is not
whether to feed comatose persons or not, but whether to care for them or to
abandon them; and that faithfully caring for comatose persons benefits them
not only by sustaining their lives but also by maintaining a moral bond, which is
far more than mere experience and feelings, of human solidarity with them.

Sometimes those who oppose caring for the comatose invoke the authority
of Pius XII, who said that gravely burdensome means of preserving life need
not be used, since a strict obligation to use them "would render the attainment
of higher, more important good too difficult. Life, health, all temporal activities
are in fact subordinated to spiritual ends."[14] But these statements of Pius XII do
not support the position of those who oppose care for the comatose. For, whatever the burdens of caring for the comatose, doing so in no way interferes with
their (or, as a rule, with anyone else's) attaining any spiritual end. And Pius XII
spoke only of situations in which the benefit of preserving life would somehow
generate some burden with respect to a higher, spiritual good. By contrast, those
who oppose caring for the comatose think that preserving the life of a comatose
person offers no benefit at all and thus cannot justify the cost of his or her care.
The premises they need are that *bodily goods are not inherent goods of persons* and that

keeping faith with the comatose is pointless. But Pius XII does not supply these premises, for he was not a dualist and he held the traditional, Judeo-Christian view of the human person and community, and of morality itself.

Some argue that the comatose are suffering from a fatal pathology, and so, if deprived of food, die because of this antecedent pathology, not because those who could provide food fail to provide it. However, this argument only shows that the decision not to feed a comatose person need not be a choice to kill him or her. It by no means shows that those who can feed the comatose have no moral obligation to do so. This point may become clearer by considering that those who have AIDS also are suffering from a fatal pathology, and without care they will die rather quickly because of it. But it does not follow that such persons may be abandoned. Similarly, the fact that comatose persons are suffering from a fatal pathology does not show that they may be abandoned, and my preceding argument, based on comparing benefits and burdens, indicates that we should not abandon them (although, of course, the benefits are less than and the burdens are different from those involved in caring for persons with AIDS).

Some assert that if it is wrong to withhold food from comatose persons, it is also wrong to withdraw or withhold from them any sort of medical treatment available to other persons; but, they argue, the latter is false; so, they conclude, it is not wrong to withhold food from the comatose. This argument can be exemplified in a form I formerly accepted with reference to Miss Karen Quinlan. Nearly everyone agrees that it was morally right to remove the respirator on which her life was thought to depend. Why, then, when the respirator was removed and she did not die, would it have been wrong to discontinue feeding her?

My present answer to this challenging question can be drawn from my preceding argument: A decision not to feed Miss Quinlan (which her father rejected with horror) would have differed greatly from the decision to remove the respirator. A decision not to feed her could have had only one or the other of two possible meanings, neither of which is morally admissible. It would have been either a choice to resolve the situation by killing her (and so would have been homicidal) or a choice to abandon her (and so, in our affluent society would have been contrary to human solidarity with her). The decision to remove her respirator might have had one of those two meanings, but in fact did not. For it could and did have another, and morally admissible, meaning: It was a choice to end the burden of *intensive* care but not to abandon her. The choice could focus exclusively on intensive care because that care by itself was both expensive and psychologically burdensome to her family, who thought that she struggled against the respirator. In general, even an affluent society such as ours must establish limits to medical treatment, and need not provide every possible treatment for persons of every condition. It is reasonable, for instance, to decide that nobody should be sustained indefinitely in an intensive care unit. Moreover, even if they are not dying, comatose and other severely mentally disabled persons stand to benefit far less from many sorts of treatment than do most other people, and it is reasonable to provide those sorts of treatment only to persons who will benefit more from them.

Admittedly, this answer does not resolve the difficult question about precisely what sorts of medical treatment should be provided to the comatose and what sorts should be withheld. However, this question is not really different from the question about how far to go in treating all those who are permanently and so severely mentally disabled that they will never (or never again) be able to do any good thing or have any good experience. For such mentally disabled persons benefit from care and treatment only as the comatose do: It keeps them alive and maintains human solidarity with them.

Notes

1. My purpose here is to try to clarify certain philosophical issues underlying the moral norm articulated in a previous collective statement: William E. May, Robert Barry, Orville Griese, et al., "Feeding and Hydrating the Permanently Unconscious and Other Vulnerable Persons," *Issues in Law & Medicine* 3(3): 203–11 (1987).

2. Even within medical circles, the language used in referring to permanently unconscious persons is bewilderingly complex, partly because the subject matter itself is not simple, partly because of the difficulties of diagnosis and prognosis, and partly because the medical community has no established tradition in the matter. On this linguistic-factual problem, see Ronald E. Cranford, "The Persistent Vegetative State: The Medical Reality (Getting the Facts Straight)," *Hastings Center Report* 18(1): 27–32 (Feb./March 1988).

3. Concerning this presupposition, see Germain Grisez and Joseph M. Boyle Jr., *Life and Death with Liberty and Justice: A Contribution to the Euthanasia Debate* (1979): 229–38.

4. See *id.* at pp. 414–22 in the context of pp. 336–414: cf. John R. Connery, "The Ethical Standards for Withholding/ Withdrawing Nutrition and Hydration," *Issues in Law & Medicine* 2(2): 87–97 (1986).

5. See David Major, "The Medical Procedures for Providing Food and Water: Indications and Effects," in Joanne Lynn, ed., *By No Extraordinary Means: The Choice to Forgo Life Sustaining Food and Water* (Bloomington, Ind.: Indiana University Press), pp. 21–28.

6. Grisez, Germain. "A Christian Ethics of Limiting Medical Treatment" in *Pope John Paul II Lecture Series in Bioethics* Vol. 2, eds. Francis Lescoe and David Liptak (Cromwell, CT: Holy Apostles Seminary, 1986), pp. 49–50.

7. See *id.*, pp. 43–44.

8. O'Rourke, Kevin, "The A.M.A. Statement on Tube Feeding: An Ethical Analysis," *America*, Nov. 22, 1986, at 322.

9. McCormick, Richard A., "The Defective Infant (2): Practical Considerations," *The Tablet* (London), July 21, 1984, at 691.

10. For a fuller philosophical and Catholic theological development of this line of argument: John Finnis, Joseph M. Boyle Jr., and Germain Grisez, *Nuclear Deterrence, Morality and Realism* (Oxford, U.K.: Oxford University Press, 1987) pp. 305–9; Germain Grisez, "Dualism and the New Morality," in 5 *Atti del Congresso Internazionale Tomasso D'Aquino nel suo Settimo Centenario* 323–30 (1977); Linacre Centre Working Party, *Euthanasia and Clinical Practice: Trends, Priorities and Alternatives* 37–43 (1982).

11. Some other articulations of the argument against dualism: Gabriel Marcel, *The Mystery of Being: Reflection and Mystery*, Vol. 1, (South Bend, IN: St. Augustine's Press, 2001), 127–53; B. A. O. Williams, "Are Persons Bodies?" in *The Philosophy of the Body: Rejections of Cartesian Dualism*, Stuart F. Spicker, ed. (New York: Times Books, 1970), 137–56; J. M. Cameron, "Bodily Existence," *Proceedings of the American Catholic Philosophical Association* 53 (1979): 59–70.

12. For an argument for free choice: Germain Grisez, Joseph M. Boyle Jr., and Olaf Tollefsen, *Free Choice: A Self-Referential Argument* (Notre Dame, IN: University of Notre Dame Press, 1976). For a philosophical articulation of an ethics in accord with the Judeo-Christian tradition, see Germain Grisez and Russell Shaw, *Beyond the New Morality: The Responsibilities of Freedom*, 3rd ed. (Notre Dame, IN: University of Notre Dame Press, 1988).

13. For fuller formulations (in some ways overstated) of these lines of argument, see Gilbert Meilaender, "On Removing Food and Water: Against the Stream," *Hastings Center Report* 14(6): 11–13 (Dec. 1984); Patrick G. Derr, "Nutrition and Hydration as Elective Therapy: Brophy and Jobes from An Ethical and Historical Perspective," *Issues in Law & Medicine* 2(1): 33–36 (1986).

14. Pius XII. "Allocution to the International Congress of Anesthesiologists," *The Pope Speaks* 4(396) (Nov. 24, 1957).

14

End-of-Life Care Revisited

Daniel P. Sulmasy, OFM

A number of claims made in recent discussions about Catholic teaching and the use of life-sustaining treatments raise important and very serious theological, philosophical, and medical questions that have received almost no direct attention or examination.

Some recent forms of argument seem to deviate from established, traditional forms of Catholic argument. Yet the nature and extent of these deviations from tradition have not been apparent to most commentators. Some recent claims have been based upon oversimplified understandings of clinical and economic reality. Still other claims appear to be based upon novel philosophies of medicine that have not been made explicit. In this brief article, I make some of these questions explicit for the sake of furthering honest discussion of the ethics of life-sustaining treatments among the faithful.

Intending Death?

Claim 1: When one discontinues the use of a feeding tube in a patient who is in a persistent vegetative state (perhaps better termed "post-coma unresponsiveness"), and that person has left no advance instructions asking that this be done for a morally legitimate reason, then one must be intending that person's death as a means of relieving his or her suffering and therefore committing euthanasia.

This form of argument has been very prominent.[1] However, there is an underlying, unrecognized premise at the argument's heart—that the proper moral principle by which to analyze the act of withdrawing a life-sustaining treatment is the rule of double effect. This rule has assumed an unprecedented prominence in Catholic circles in recent years, due to the influence of what has been called the "New Natural Law Theory." According to this theory, which effectively removes ontological considerations from natural-law thinking, everyone must act for one of a small number of reasons called "basic goods," and one may never act directly against one of these basic goods. These theorists recognize that, in real life, however, one is constantly facing choices in which one good must be sacrificed so that another can be realized.

According to this theory, one may tolerate an act that goes against a basic good (e.g., undermines respect for life or marriage) only if this bad result is an indirect, unintended side effect of acting to promote another basic good. That is to say, the rule of double effect applies in all these situations. Therefore, in a feeding tube case, the New Natural Law Theory directs the patient's loved ones to ask themselves, "What good am I trying to accomplish here?" If they answer, "Relieving the patient's suffering," they will violate the rule of double effect. Since the feeding tube itself does not appear to be doing any harm, the only way to relieve the suffering of the patient is by way of making the patient dead. Therefore, it is concluded that the act is morally impermissible.

However, the story is complicated because commentators who would require feeding tubes for patients suffering from post-coma unresponsiveness are not the only ones who use the rule of double effect in this situation. Some who argue that it is permissible to withdraw feeding tubes from such patients also invoke the rule of double effect in doing so. To make the argument work, however, they are forced to conclude that the treatment is of "no benefit," so that even the most minimal burdens caused by the feeding tube can be considered disproportionate. Of note, this seems to entail the judgment that life itself is not a good, since the effect of the treatment (maintaining life) is judged to be of no benefit. Justifiably, this has upset orthodox Catholic sensibilities, since it seems to denigrate the value of human life.

I argue, however, that both sides of the debate are mistaken because they have framed the problem using the wrong principle. The Catholic moral tradition has for several centuries relied upon the casuistry of withholding and withdrawing extraordinary means of care as the proper framework for analyzing such cases, not the rule of double effect. The moral theology of forgoing extraordinary means of care was developed independently of the rule of double effect and this rule was never invoked in its development or justification. Instead, the traditional understanding of forgoing extraordinary means has been based upon the principles of "physical and moral impossibility."

These principles are based upon the understanding that although negative precepts ("do not commit adultery") bind absolutely, positive precepts ("fast on Ash Wednesday") are always limited in a finite world. They are limited by physical impossibility (what cannot be done) and so-called moral impossibility (that which is beyond what a reasonable person can be expected to do or to bear in carrying out a duty). The intention of a person who refrains from fasting (say, because of age or infirmity) is not to denigrate the value of penance and self-mortification; it is, rather, to say, "I have done all that the Lord requires of me, given my finite physical, psychological, social, financial, and spiritual resources. Fasting is beyond me, and I can forgo this otherwise obligatory duty."

The forgoing of extraordinary means of care emerges from this form of moral analysis. One has a positive duty to sustain one's life, but this duty is limited. One need not do everything conceivable to sustain one's life. And when a person forgoes a life-sustaining treatment under this analysis, one cannot conclude that that person has the intention of causing death.

When a faithful Catholic withholds or withdraws a life-sustaining treatment, the moral object of the act, the intention-in-acting, is to forgo a treatment that is demanding more than one can reasonably be expected to bear. The intention is fulfilled when the treatment is stopped. In so doing, one foresees death following, but death is not within the scope of one's intention. Whereas the outer limits of judgments about when this is permissible are determined by the community of believers, decisions about what is extraordinary will always depend upon the individual case—the constitution of the patient as a person integrally considered; the nature of the condition and its treatment; and the clinical, social, and economic conditions, among others.

The traditional criteria for judging that a treatment is extraordinary (i.e., morally optional) have been either that it is futile (physical impossibility) or that it is more burdensome than beneficial (moral impossibility). Burdens have included not just pain but also the broad range of physical, psychological, intellectual, financial, social, and spiritual resources of the person, including such traditional notions as horror or repugnance at the state in which one will be left by the treatment (e.g., after amputation).

Some commentators have argued that the ordinary/extraordinary means distinction is merely an application of the rule of double effect, but this is not true historically, and in fact makes no sense when applied to many situations in which there is clear consensus among the faithful that treatment would be "extraordinary" or morally optional.

One important difference is that, under the rule of double effect, only the positive and negative effects associated with the action itself count in the proportionality assessment. When this is applied to withdrawing life-sustaining treatments, this means that the only benefits and burdens that count are those bad effects caused by the withdrawal of the treatment (e.g., shortening life) and the benefits resulting from stopping the treatment (e.g., relieving pain and side effects caused by the treatment itself and capping the treatment's costs). This sets an almost impossibly high standard. Unless death is just minutes away, the treatment itself would need to be torturous to the patient for one to view its withdrawal as a good proportionate to the bad effect of shortening something of so great a value as life itself. However, under the analysis proposed by the extraordinary-means tradition, the burdens of the disease itself, not just the burdens of the treatment, count in the proportionality considerations.

For example, Cardinal John De Lugo wrote in the seventeenth century that one had no obligation to prolong one's life by dousing oneself with water if one were being burned to death and water were reasonably available, but only in a supply great enough to prolong one's burning to death, not enough to extinguish the fire. The pain caused by the condition itself (i.e., being on fire), which the treatment (water) only prolonged, and not just the suffering caused by water itself (which in this case is not a burden but rather a source of temporary relief) counted in the evaluation of benefits and burdens.

Many commentators who analyze cases of the withdrawal of life-sustaining treatments under the rule of double effect appear to overestimate the burdens caused directly by treatments such as ventilators. This is the only way they could use this rule to justify the claim that the positive effects of withdrawal are proportionate to the negative effect of shortening life. This might work theoretically, but in real life most life-sustaining treatments do not themselves cause much suffering. Rather, they tend to relieve some symptoms and to prolong the suffering associated with the underlying condition—much like the water in Cardinal De Lugo's case.

For example, if a patient is comatose, he or she will not feel the discomfort of having an endotracheal tube. So the directly intended good effect of stopping the ventilator cannot be the relief of the suffering caused by the ventilator. If the patient is awake, the discomfort of ventilation is often preferable to feeling the discomfort of shortness of breath. In both cases, it is generally the suffering caused by the *disease*, not its treatment, that constitutes the true burden. Thus, under double-effect analysis, stopping the ventilator in most cases will be euthanasia since the aim would appear to be to relieve the patient from a state of suffering that is being prolonged by the machine. The only way this could be accomplished would be by means of making the patient dead, and so it would not be allowed.

However, according to the traditional Catholic analysis, stopping ventilator treatment in a patient dying of a painful cancer would be the morally permissible forgoing of an extraordinary means of care. The burdens of the disease count in the equation (e.g., the pain caused by the cancer). The intention is not to make the patient dead, but to stop a treatment at a point at which the burdens of the disease and its treatment are greater than what one could reasonably be expected to bear in carrying out one's duty to preserve one's life.

Extraordinary Means: Whose Point of View?

According to the traditional Catholic analysis (which was developed centuries before the legal concept of substituted judgment was invented), when family members or religious superiors make a judgment for the patient, they are acting on the patient's behalf and assuming the patient's point of view. The tradition has never focused on the family's motives and beliefs as the central moral concern. The proposed analysis that some are now urging changes this, however, by making the central moral question, when patients cannot speak for themselves, "What basic good is the family member attempting to realize by way of his or her act?" The Catholic tradition, by contrast, asks the family to assess whether the patient could be presumed to have met the reasonable limits of what would be necessary in carrying out his or her duty to preserve the gift of life. This difference is so subtle that it largely goes unnoticed, but in reality the shift is monumental, and changes the whole character of the analysis.

The Cost of Care

To complicate matters further, the way that claims about the financial costs of treatments have been bandied about in recent discussions appears to draw upon an insufficient understanding of the actual clinical and economic reality. Traditional analysis has allowed consideration of costs to enter into judgments about whether treatments are extraordinary either because (a) the patient has decided to forgo a treatment as an act of charity or (b) because the treatment is prohibitively expensive. But recent discussions seem dominated by a somewhat oversimplified understanding of the costs of certain types of treatment. Tube feeding is assumed to be cheap. However, tube feeding involves far more than the cost of the nutrient solution.

First, little attention is paid to the fact that no one ever gets to the point of being in postcoma unresponsiveness without millions of dollars having already been spent in hopes of a recovery. It takes six months of intensive care just to make the diagnosis! Second, the additional costs of caring for patients—such as special beds, nursing care, supplies, testing, pumps, electricity, hospitalizations for complications, and so forth—are never considered in discussions of the costs involved in supplying tube feeding.

On the other side of the equation, many treatments that seem more technologically sophisticated than tube feeding have become much less expensive than many commentators seem to appreciate. It has been estimated that the annual cost of feeding tube supplies for home treatment (adjusted to 2005 dollars) is about $12,000 per year.[2] This is relatively cheap, but it does not count any costs for nursing home care (which would bring the cost to $868,000 per year[3]), nor does it count the labor costs if treatment were given at home (estimated at $37,000 per year[4]). This is roughly comparable to the annual cost of continuous ambulatory peritoneal dialysis (CAPD) at home, which is about $17,000 per year for supplies[5]; $28,000 if one includes labor, electricity, testing, and other factors.[6]

Some developing countries such as Malaysia have reduced the annual cost of the supplies for CAPD to as little as $7,000.[7] Both tube feeding and CAPD can be done at home. Both involve placing a tube through the abdominal wall to replace a lost physiological function. Patients die in similar time frames after discontinuing dialysis or feeding tubes (about two weeks).

If one of the main arguments in favor of declaring feeding by tube to be ordinary and obligatory is its low cost relative to other treatments and relative to the wealth of developed nations, then CAPD would also have to be considered in principle ordinary and morally obligatory for all patients in renal failure, even those suffering from postcoma unresponsiveness. Similarly, ventilators can now be used at home, oxygen can be delivered via oxygen concentrators, and the price of this treatment is thought to have come down considerably from the $77,000 per year estimated in 1997.[8] A year's worth of antiretroviral drugs for HIV costs substantially more than this.

The point is that the church must be extremely careful about the reasoning being invoked to conclude that feeding tubes are ordinary and morally obligatory in any particular clinical circumstance. It does not seem to me that the magisterium has explicitly decided to revoke a six-hundred-year-old tradition of moral reasoning in favor of a new method for analyzing such cases. And if this new method of analysis is used in the case of feeding tubes, the precedent-setting implications are potentially astounding, given the propensity for life-sustaining treatments to become increasingly available and less expensive relative to the economies of the developed world. A rash move in this case threatens to make Catholics servants of technology, when the point of technology ought to be its service to the human person.

The Nature of Human Suffering

Claim 2A: It cannot be argued that, if patients are in the condition of postcoma unresponsiveness, feeding tubes cause them any pain. Since, by virtue of their brain damage, such patients cannot be said to suffer from the treatment, the only intention one could have in discontinuing feeding-tube treatment would be to make them dead by way of a judgment that they are unworthy of life.

Claim 2B: If their feeding tubes are discontinued, patients in postcoma unresponsiveness suffer miserably from the pangs of starvation and die with parched tongues and cracked, bleeding lips. It is cruel and inhumane to make a person suffer so.

Recent arguments about the use of feeding tubes in patients who suffer from postcoma unresponsiveness raise significant questions about the nature of suffering, the human person, and Catholic teaching. Some people, in arguing that feeding tubes are always ordinary and morally obligatory in cases of postcoma unresponsiveness, have used both of the arguments above. The arguments do not appear in the same paragraph, but have been invoked by the same source. When they are placed side by side, it is easier to see that these arguments are internally inconsistent. One cannot argue both that tube feeding must be continued because such patients lack the neurological substratum for experiencing suffering and also that tube feeding cannot be discontinued because the patients will thereby experience intense suffering.

Additionally, the clinical descriptions of such deaths are medically misguided. Most persons who die of chronic illnesses stop eating at the end of life, and dehydration is generally a contributing cause of such deaths, whether resulting from cancer or tuberculosis. While there is a tendency towards dry mouth (often exacerbated by the injudicious use of oxygen), this problem can be treated with ice chips, sips of water, or gentle mouth swabbing by nurses or family members.

Also, it is unclear whether feeding tubes help relieve the sensation of hunger. They provide no taste or smell or oral sensation, and since the nutritional solution is usually dripped into the tube continually to avoid the side effect of aspiration pneumonia, feeding tubes do not provide a sensation of satiety—the patient's stomach is never full. Thus, discontinuing the tube would not deprive a patient of a sensation of satiety. Finally, the question exists whether any of these physical sensations can be cognitively appreciated by a patient who lacks function in the cortex of the brain.

But such contradictions and clinical mischaracterizations aside, these arguments raise much deeper and serious questions for Catholics about the nature of human suffering. Do we believe that a person in postcoma unresponsiveness cannot suffer? Provided that the diagnosis is relatively certain, it would seem that there could be no cognitive appreciation of such sensations as pain or thirst. But does this mean that the patient is not suffering? Certainly, in ordinary English, it would appear grammatically correct to say that a person is *suffering* from postcoma unresponsiveness. And no sane person would ever say that he or she wished to be in such a condition. But if a person, integrally considered, is in a state in which he or she is deprived of conscious interaction with the physical world, but not yet dead and united with the One, True, and Eternal Source of all life and all goodness—is this person not in a state of suffering?

As Pope John Paul II wrote in *Salvifici Doloris*:

Suffering is something which is *still wider* than sickness, more complex and at the same time still more deeply rooted in humanity itself. A certain idea of this problem comes to us from the distinction between physical suffering and moral suffering. This distinction is based upon the double dimension of the human being and indicates the bodily and spiritual element as the immediate or direct subject of suffering. Insofar as the words "suffering" and "pain," can, up to a certain degree, be used as synonyms, *physical suffering* is present when "the body is hurting" in some way, whereas *moral suffering* is "pain of the soul." In fact, it is a question of pain of a spiritual nature, and not only of the "psychological" dimension of pain which accompanies both moral and physical suffering. The vastness and the many forms of moral suffering are certainly no less in number than the forms of physical suffering.[9]

It would seem that the church, when considering the use of life-sustaining treatments in patients with postcoma unresponsiveness, must be particularly careful about making judgments that depend upon assumptions about the nature of human suffering that might narrow the field of what we, as Christians, understand about the nature of human suffering. We must, above all, never endorse the notion that any of the essential features of human beings can be reduced to brain states. Persons who suffer, suffer as persons in their totality.

What Is a "Medical" Act?

Claim 3: The use of feeding tubes is an act of basic human caring, and is not a medical act.

This argument is commonly invoked by those who would declare feeding tubes in postcoma unresponsiveness an *a priori* ordinary means and therefore, in principle, morally obligatory. However, one can raise serious questions about whether this line of argument can bear the freight that has been loaded upon it.

It is obvious that feeding is associated with caring, beginning with the relationship between mother and child. Eating is associated with love in the Scriptures, from the multiplication of the loaves and fishes to the postresurrection appearances of Jesus at Emmaus and shores of Lake Tiberius. And it is clear that the emotional significance of feeding tubes, and their symbolism, make the decision to withhold or withdraw feeding tubes particularly stressful for family members, even compared with the stress of forgoing other treatments.

No one doubts that only a physician can perform a percutaneous endoscopic gastrostomy (PEG) and insert a tube to be used for feeding. In this sense, it is clearly a medical act. Some argue, however, that once the tube is in place, its use becomes nonmedical, obligatory, ordinary care.

This argument deserves more attention than has been given to it.

First, logically, this would imply that withholding a PEG tube would be morally permissible, since its *insertion* is a medical act, whereas discontinuing its use once it is in place would be prohibited, since its *use* is *not* a medical act. This would be the first instance of a Catholic teaching that there is a morally relevant distinction between withholding and withdrawing care. The tradition has always consistently held that the same criteria apply to withholding as apply to withdrawing life-sustaining treatments. This would be another departure from tradition.

Second, there seems to be, on the basis of this argument alone, no principled reason for distinguishing between postcoma unresponsiveness and any other clinical condition. It would seem that one ought to be prohibited from discontinuing assisted hydration and nutrition for any and all patients if the act is not medical and represents basic human care. If this intervention is necessary in order to show respect for the dignity of the person who suffers from postcoma unresponsiveness, then it also ought to be given to other patients who have no less dignity and are no less worthy of similar respect. This, of course, would have the absurd conclusion that no one dying of a chronic illness could have a feeding tube withdrawn.

Third, unless it is totally ad hoc, the general form of the argument being advocated here must be something like the following: that whenever a medical device has been inserted or attached to a patient, and a layperson can be trained to use it, the use of the device becomes nonmedical and in principle ordinary and morally obligatory once the procedure has been completed. Under this argument, a person who had undergone a leg amputation and the attachment of a prosthetic limb would be obliged to use that prosthetic limb and crutches even if his or her other leg were later amputated because of life-threatening gangrene. It would be wrong, according to the argument, to forgo the use of the prosthesis in order to accept life in a wheelchair. Even though, given the new condition, using a wheelchair might be much easier and would render the patient more mobile, the use of the prosthesis and crutches would be required because the use of the prosthesis had become nonmedical and morally obligatory. Such a conclusion seems odd in the light of common sense and Catholic tradition.

So perhaps the form of the argument should be modified in such a way that the medical device in question would have to be life-sustaining in order to be declared nonmedical and morally obligatory. But then support with a home ventilator would, in principle, be considered nonmedical and morally obligatory and could never be discontinued because, as with a feeding tube, although the ventilator's use might be initiated through a medical act, it can be used by laypeople trained for that purpose, it is attached to the person, and it is life-sustaining. Yet since the time of Pope Pius XII, the paradigmatic example of a potentially extraordinary means of care has been the ventilator. Therefore, this cannot be the correct form of the argument either.

So perhaps the argument must be amended to say that the act becomes nonmedical when the substance delivered to the patient by a layperson via an indwelling device is something all human beings need in order to survive. Again, however, this formulation will not distinguish a ventilator from a feeding tube since, at least in some cases, the gas-exchange capacity of a ventilated patient remains normal and it is only the ability to breathe that is impaired, so the patient is treated with room air via the ventilator. Everyone needs air. Therefore, unless the ventilator is supplying additional oxygen, it could never be considered extraordinary and could never be stopped. And once again, this fails to square with the *sensus fidelium*.

Perhaps one might construct the argument so that an act becomes nonmedical when the substance delivered to the patient by a layperson via an indwelling device is something that all human beings commonly need in order to survive *and* one that can be delivered to the patient without using any additional device. This might appear to distinguish the ventilator from the feeding tube. But this argument will not work either. One needs at least a syringe to deliver the nutrition via a PEG tube, and if the patient cannot breathe, one needs at least an Ambu bag (Ambu is the trademarked name of a self-reinflating bag used in resuscitation) to deliver air to the patient. The need for an extra device would not distinguish medically assisted nutrition from medically assisted ventilation.

As a last resort, one might ask: What if the trached patient were able to breathe on his own—would you remove the oxygen from the room? The answer is clearly no; that would be a direct act of killing. Taking away someone's supply of oxygen is not analogous to a failure to provide food. The killing/allowing to die distinction classifies the former as killing and the latter as allowing to die.[10]

Taking the oxygen out of the air that a dying person is breathing is killing and is always wrong. Failing to provide food is allowing to die. Doing so is sometimes wrong and sometimes morally permissible. It is wrong not to feed a baby who can eat. It is not wrong to refrain from force-feeding someone dying of cancer who has lost his appetite.

The proper parallel is not between air and food but between breathing and swallowing. The analogous medico–moral issues concern the interventions aimed at assisting persons who have lost these functions. If that is so, then just as there are reasonable limits to the obligation one has to replace the lost function of breathing via a ventilator machine or an Ambu bag, there are limits to the obligation one has to replace a lost ability to swallow with a pump machine or a syringe. So there seems to be no principled way to define a medical act in such a way that feeding tubes are classified as "nonmedical" while other treatment modalities that are initiated and prescribed by physicians remain classified as "medical."

In any event, why does this odd foray into an idiosyncratic interpretation of the philosophy of medicine require a dogmatic definition from the church? The concepts of "health," "disease," "therapy," and "medicine" are also hotly debated in the philosophy of medicine. Is the answer to the medical/nonmedical question of such import that the church must define which acts are, when performed by medical personnel, in fact not medical?

Perhaps more importantly, the whole argument is irrelevant from the point of view of traditional Catholic teaching. The tradition has never considered the question of whether something was "medical" to be a criterion for distinguishing ordinary from extraordinary means of care. Very commonplace acts, such as traveling to a healthier climate, eating certain kinds of foods, or even eating itself have all have been considered, in the proper circumstances, "extraordinary means" under traditional analysis. Does the church think it is important (a) to define this distinction between the medical and the nonmedical and then (b) to alter the tradition and make this a decisive factor in distinguishing ordinary from extraordinary means of care?

Does the symbolic value of a feeding tube itself carry the weight of the argument? Is the symbolic meaning of eating in the Gospels carried by the physiology of nutrient absorption, or by the interpersonal human experience we normally consider part of sharing a meal? What would the implications of such a dogmatic declaration be for our Eucharistic practices? Would we thereby say, of a person who cannot swallow but is awake and alert, that it would be preferable to deliver a small bit of the consecrated bread or wine into the feeding tube than to place a drop of the consecrated wine on the person's tongue? Which would we consider truer to the sacramental meaning of sharing in the Body and Blood of Christ? These questions ought to be carefully considered before any formal dogmatic pronouncements are made concerning the use of feeding tubes.

Serious Examination Is Needed

In this brief article, I have considered several underlying questions raised by recent discussions about life-sustaining treatments within the church. These are not the surface questions that have dominated media coverage, political lobbying, and polemical discourse about these issues. In my judgment, these questions require serious examination in advance of any formal dogmatic resolution of these hotly disputed questions.

Notes

1. The arguments outlined in this section are presented in much greater detail in Daniel P. Sulmasy, "End of Life Care and the Rule of Double Effect: Some Clarifications and Distinctions," *Vera Lex*, 6 (1 & 2).

2. P. Reddy and M. Malone, "Cost and Outcome Analysis of Home Parenteral and Enteral Nutrition," *Journal of Parenteral and Enteral Nutrition*, 22(5): 302–10.

3. Susan L. Mitchell, et al., "Tube-Feeding versus Hand-Feeding Nursing Home Residents with Advanced Dementia: A Cost Comparison," *Journal of the American Medical Directors Association* (supplement), 5(2): S22–S29.

4. Melvin Heyman, et al., "Economic and Psychologic Costs for Maternal Caregivers of Gastrostomy-Dependent Children," *Journal of Pediatrics*, 45(4): 511–16.

5. A. F. De Vecchi, M. Dratwa, and M. E. Wiedemann, "Healthcare Systems and End-Stage Renal Disease (ESRD) Therapies—An International Review: Costs and Reimbursement/Funding of ESRD Therapies," *Nephrology Dialysis Transplantation* (supplement), 14(6): 31–41.

6. David W. Johnson, et al., "Cost-Savings from Peritoneal Dialysis Therapy Time Extension Using Icodextrin," *Advances in Peritoneal Dialysis*, 19(2003): 81–85.

7. Lai Seong Hooi, et al., "Economic Evaluation of Centre Haemodialysis and Continuous Ambulatory Peritoneal Dialysis in Ministry of Health Hospitals, Malaysia," *Nephrology*, 10(1): 25–32.

8. Mary A. Sevick and Douglas D. Bradham, "Economic Value of Caregiver Effort in Maintaining Long-Term Ventilator-Assisted Individuals at Home," *Heart & Lung*, 26(2): 148–57.

9. John Paul II, *Salvifici Doloris*, 1984, section 5, available at www.vatican.va/holy_father/john_paul_ii/apost_letters/documents/hf_jp-ii_apl _11021984_salvifici-doloris_en.html.

10. Daniel P. Sulmasy, "Killing and Allowing to Die: Another Look," *Journal of Law, Medicine & Ethics*, 26(1): 55–64.

PART FIVE

John Paul II's Papal Allocution and Responses

On March 20, 2004, Pope John Paul II addressed participants in an international congress at the Vatican on "Life-Sustaining Treatments and Vegetative State: Scientific Advances and Ethical Dilemmas." The pope's speech, "Care for Patients in a 'Permanent' Vegetative State," set off a vigorous debate, especially in the United States, regarding its authority as well as how the speech should be interpreted, and it also intensified the debate about the moral justifiability of forgoing or withdrawing artificial nutrition and hydration for patients in PVS. The papal allocution seems to have affirmed the position that began to emerge in the early 1980s, namely, that artificial nutrition and hydration are a form of basic care and therefore are generally morally obligatory. This section presents the text of the papal allocution and a range of responses to it.

The papal allocution gave rise to several critical questions. Does the allocution, in fact, represent a shift in traditional Catholic teaching on forgoing or withdrawing life-sustaining treatment? If it does, what are the shifts? If it does not, why is that the case (i.e., how is it in continuity with the tradition)? Does the allocution require that artificial nutrition and hydration always be employed for patients in PVS? If not, under which circumstances may they not be employed? Does the pope's teaching about artificial nutrition and hydration apply only to patients in PVS or, a fortiori, does it apply to all patients? What is the authority of the allocution? Does it once and for all settle the debate about discontinuing artificial nutrition and hydration in PVS patients and other severely brain-damaged patients? What are implications of the allocution for Catholic health care and for the care of patients in Catholic health care facilities? What are implications for honoring advance directives?

Other questions focus on the allocution's assumptions or specific claims within the allocution. For example, is PVS a severe disability or a fatal pathology? Are the scientific claims in this speech adequately based, especially those regarding misdiagnoses, recovery from PVS, and the ability of PVS patients to experience pain and suffering? Is life itself a benefit even if it cannot be experienced by the patient? Is it actually the case that discontinuing artificial nutrition and hydration can only be euthanasia by omission? In one way or another, the articles in this section address many of these questions. And, as one might expect, the positions of the authors vary considerably.

15

Care for Patients in a "Permanent" Vegetative State

Pope John Paul II

1. I cordially greet all of you who took part in the International Congress: "Life-Sustaining Treatments and Vegetative State: Scientific Advances and Ethical Dilemmas." I wish to extend a special greeting to Bishop Elio Sgreccia, vice president of the Pontifical Academy for Life, and to Professor Gian Luigi Gigli, president of the International Federation of Catholic Medical Associations and selfless champion of the fundamental value of life, who has kindly expressed your shared feelings.

This important congress, organized jointly by the Pontifical Academy for Life and the International Federation of Catholic Medical Associations, is dealing with a very significant issue: the clinical condition called the *vegetative state*. The complex scientific, ethical, social, and pastoral implications of such a condition require in-depth reflections and a fruitful interdisciplinary dialogue, as evidenced by the intense and carefully structured program of your work sessions.

2. With deep esteem and sincere hope, the church encourages the efforts of men and women of science who, sometimes at great sacrifice, daily dedicate their task of study and research to the improvement of the diagnostic, therapeutic, prognostic, and rehabilitative possibilities confronting those patients who rely completely on those who care for and assist them. The person in a vegetative state, in fact, shows no evident sign of self-awareness or of awareness of the environment and seems unable to interact with others or to react to specific stimuli.

Scientists and researchers realize that one must, first of all, arrive at a correct diagnosis, which usually requires prolonged and careful observation in specialized centers, given also the high number of diagnostic errors reported in the literature. Moreover, not a few of these persons, with appropriate treatment and with specific rehabilitation programs, have been able to emerge from a vegetative state. On the contrary, many others unfortunately remain prisoners of their condition even for long stretches of time and without needing technological support.

In particular, the term *permanent vegetative state* has been coined to indicate the condition of those patients whose "vegetative state" continues for over a year. Actually, there is no different diagnosis that corresponds to such a definition, but only a conventional prognostic judgment relative to the fact that the recovery of patients statistically speaking is ever more difficult as the condition of vegetative state is prolonged in time.

However, we must neither forget nor underestimate that there are well-documented cases of at least partial recovery even after many years; we can thus state that medical science up until now is still unable to predict with certainty who among patients in this condition will recover and who will not.

3. Faced with patients in similar clinical conditions, there are some who cast doubt on the persistence of the "human quality" itself, almost as if the adjective *vegetative* (whose use is now solidly established), which symbolically describes a clinical state, could or should be instead applied to the sick as such, actually demeaning their value and personal dignity. In this sense it must be noted that this term, even when confined to the clinical context, is certainly not the most felicitous when applied to human beings.

In opposition to such trends of thought, I feel the duty to reaffirm strongly that the intrinsic value and personal dignity of every human being do not change no matter what the concrete circumstances of his or her life. A man, even if seriously ill or disabled in the exercise of his highest functions, is and always will be a man, and he will never become a "vegetable" or an "animal."

Even our brothers and sisters who find themselves in the clinical condition of a "vegetative state" retain their human dignity in all its fullness. The loving gaze of God the Father continues to fall upon them, acknowledging them as his sons and daughters, especially in need of help.

4. Medical doctors and health care personnel, society and the church have moral duties toward these persons from which they cannot exempt themselves

without lessening the demands both of professional ethics and human and Christian solidarity.

The sick person in a vegetative state, awaiting recovery or a natural end, still has the right to basic health care (nutrition, hydration, cleanliness, warmth, etc.), and to the prevention of complications related to his confinement to bed. He also has the right to appropriate rehabilitative care and to be monitored for clinical signs of eventual recovery.

I should like particularly to underline how the administration of water and food, even when provided by artificial means, always represents a natural means of preserving life, not a medical act. Its use, furthermore, should be considered in principle ordinary and proportionate, and as such morally obligatory insofar as and until it is seen to have attained its proper finality, which in the present case consists in providing nourishment to the patient and alleviation of his suffering.

The obligation to provide the "normal care due to the sick in such cases" (Congregation for the Doctrine of the Faith, Declaration on Euthanasia, p. IV) includes, in fact, the use of nutrition and hydration (cf. Pontifical Council *Cor Unum, Dans le cadre*, 2.4.4; Pontifical Council for Pastoral Assistance to Health Care Workers, *Charter of Health Care Workers*, No. 120). The evaluation of probabilities, founded on waning hopes for recovery when the vegetative state is prolonged beyond a year, cannot ethically justify the cessation or interruption of minimal care for the patient, including nutrition and hydration. Death by starvation or dehydration is in fact the only possible outcome as a result of their withdrawal. In this sense it ends up becoming, if done knowingly and willingly, true and proper euthanasia by omission.

In this regard, I recall what I wrote in the encyclical *Evangelium vitae*, making it clear that "by *euthanasia* in the true and proper sense must be understood an action or omission that by its very nature and intention brings about death, with the purpose of eliminating all pain"; such an act is always "a serious violation of the law of God, since it is the deliberate and morally unacceptable killing of a human person" (No. 65). Besides, the moral principle is well known according to which even the simple doubt of being in the presence of a living person already imposes the obligation of full respect and of abstaining from any act that aims at anticipating the person's death.

5. Considerations about the "quality of life," often actually dictated by psychological, social and economic pressures, cannot take precedence over general principles.

First of all, no evaluation of costs can outweigh the value of the fundamental good which we are trying to protect, that of human life. Moreover, to admit that decisions regarding man's life can be based on the external acknowledgment of its quality is the same as acknowledging that increasing and decreasing levels of quality of life, and therefore of human dignity, can be attributed from an external perspective to any subject, thus introducing into social relations a discriminatory and eugenic principle.

Moreover, it is not possible to rule out a priori that the withdrawal of nutrition and hydration, as reported by authoritative studies, is the source of considerable suffering for the sick person even if we can see only the reactions at the level of the autonomic nervous system or of gestures. Modern clinical neurophysiology and neuroimaging techniques, in fact, seem to point to the lasting quality in these patients of elementary forms of communication and analysis of stimuli.

6. However, it is not enough to reaffirm the general principle according to which the value of a man's life cannot be made subordinate to any judgment of its quality expressed by other men; it is necessary to promote the taking of positive actions as a stand against pressures to withdraw hydration and nutrition as a way to put an end to the lives of these patients.

It is necessary, above all, to support those families who have had one of their loved ones struck down by this terrible clinical condition. They cannot be left alone with their heavy human, psychological and financial burden. Although the care for these patients is not in general particularly costly, society must allot sufficient resources for the care of this sort of frailty, by way of bringing about appropriate concrete initiatives such as, for example, the creation of a network of awakening centers with specialized treatment and rehabilitation programs; financial support and home assistance for families when patients are moved back home at the end of intensive rehabilitation programs; the establishment of facilities which can accommodate those cases in which there is no family able to deal with the problem or to provide "breaks" for those families who are at risk of psychological and moral burnout.

Proper care for these patients and their families should, moreover, include the presence and the witness of a medical doctor and an entire team, who are asked to help the family understand that they are there as allies who are in this struggle with them. The participation of volunteers represents a basic support to enable the family to break out of its isolation and to help it to realize that it is a precious and not a forsaken part of the social fabric.

In these situations, then, spiritual counseling and pastoral aid are particularly important as help for recovering the deepest meaning of an apparently desperate condition.

7. Distinguished ladies and gentlemen, in conclusion I exhort you as men and women of science responsible for the dignity of the medical profession to guard jealously the principle according to which the true task of medicine is "to cure if possible, always to care."

As a pledge and support of this, your authentic humanitarian mission to give comfort and support to your suffering brothers and sisters, I remind you of the words of Jesus: "Amen, I say to you, whatever you did for one of these least brothers of mine, you did for me" (Mt. 25:40).

In this light I invoke upon you the assistance of him whom a meaningful saying of the church fathers describes as *Christus medicus*, and in entrusting your work to the protection of Mary, consoler of the sick and comforter of the dying, I lovingly bestow on all of you a special apostolic blessing.

16

John Paul II on the "Vegetative State"

Richard M. Doerflinger

In a March 20 address, Pope John Paul II made a very significant contribution to an ethical debate that has troubled Catholic ethicists in the United States and elsewhere for many years: The feeding of patients diagnosed as being in a "vegetative" state.

His speech was addressed to participants in an international congress titled "Life-Sustaining Treatments and Vegetative State: Scientific Advances and Ethical Dilemmas," co-sponsored by the Pontifical Academy for Life and the International Federation of Catholic Medical Associations. The congress was attended by physicians, scientists, ethicists, and others from over forty countries.

The Holy Father's address touched upon at least four aspects of this issue.

Main Points

First, a statement of theological anthropology. Against all who would deny the inherent worth and human dignity of persons in a vegetative state, the Holy Father strongly affirmed that

> the intrinsic value and personal dignity of every human being do not change, no matter what the concrete circumstances of his or her life. *A man, even if seriously ill or disabled in the exercise of his highest functions, is and always will be a man,* and he will never become a "vegetable" or an "animal." Even our brothers and sisters who

find themselves in the clinical condition of a "vegetative state" retain their human dignity in all its fullness. (n. 3, original emphasis)

Second, a recognition of the latest medical and scientific findings on the vegetative state, reviewed at length during the congress itself. Misdiagnosis of the vegetative state is common, prognoses (including predictions that patients can never recover) are far from reliable, and the assumption that this state of unresponsiveness entails complete absence of internal sensation or awareness is being seriously questioned.

Third, a statement of medical ethics. Patients in this state deserve the normal care that is due all patients out of respect for their human dignity, including nutrition and hydration.

I should like particularly to underline how the administration of water and food, even when provided by artificial means, always represents a *natural means* of preserving life, not a *medical act*. Its use, furthermore, should be considered, in principle, *ordinary and proportionate*, and as such morally obligatory, insofar as and until it is seen to have attained its proper finality, which in the present case consists in providing nourishment to the patient and alleviation of his suffering. (n. 4, original emphasis)

Fourth, a statement of social ethics. Families caring for patients in this state should not be abandoned to suffer alone but must receive all possible support from society, including appropriate "respite care" and other practical help.

Many ethicists will focus on the third statement, which makes a stronger and more explicit statement in favor of providing food and fluids to these patients than has been seen from authoritative Vatican sources. To ignore the other elements of the Holy Father's address, however, would wrench this specific norm out of its context in a profound theology of the human person, an understanding of the latest scientific data, and a heroic social ethic demanding that the burdens of caring for the most helpless should be borne by all.

Affirmation of Human Dignity

Three questions have been at the heart of Catholic moral debate on providing food and fluids to the patient in a vegetative state. Does the life of such a patient have the same inherent value and dignity as the lives of others, placing essentially the same moral demands on us for care despite the person's low "quality of life"?

Is such a state generally to be seen as a severe condition of disability demanding assistance from others, rather than as a "terminal" illness which morally can be allowed to run its course toward death? Is artificially assisted food and fluids to be seen as a form of "normal care" care owed in principle to all patients?[1] The Holy Father answers all these questions in the affirmative.

His insistence on the full value and dignity of these patient's lives, and his warning against external judgments attributing "increasing and decreasing levels of quality of life, and therefore of human dignity," to patients, seems a direct response to a theory held by many theologians in the United States for some years. According to that theory, there is generally no moral obligation to sustain the life of a patient in a vegetative state, even by food and fluids, because such a patient can no longer pursue the "spiritual purposes" to which human life is ordered; to feed and maintain this patient indefinitely only preserves a "biological existence" incapable of engaging in human acts. In the March 20 speech, by contrast, the decisive fact is the patient's inherent dignity as a human being and his or her status as a child of God, in need of care and support—not the kinds of acts that may make a life seem worthwhile to an outside observer.

The "spiritual purposes" standard for withdrawing food and fluids has been challenged before. In 1992, after two years of research and drafting, the U.S. bishops' Committee for Pro-Life Activities issued a resource paper titled "Nutrition and Hydration: Moral and Pastoral Reflections."[2] The paper concluded that withholding or withdrawing medically assisted nutrition and hydration is a form of euthanasia by omission when the intent is to end life. It found that nutrition and hydration are generally a form of "ordinary care," or at least an ordinary means of sustaining life, because they are basic needs which are effective in sustaining life (except for the imminently dying patient) and do not often impose grave burdens on the patient. The paper warned against the use of "quality of life" judgments to dismiss the value of disabled patients' lives. Finally, while recognizing that theological debate would continue, it found the "spiritual purposes" theory unconvincing, instead recommending a presumption in favor of assisted feeding for patients in the vegetative state.

The 1992 paper's general conclusions were reflected in the 1995 revision of the U.S. bishops' *Ethical and Religious Directives for Catholic Health Care Services* which govern practice in Catholic health facilities. That edition, and the 2001 revision now in effect, state: "There should be a presumption in favor of providing nutrition and hydration to all patients, including patients who require medically assisted nutrition and hydration, as long as this is of sufficient benefit to

outweigh the burdens involved to the patient" (directive 58). And in 1998, the
Holy Father singled out the Pro-Life Committee's paper for praise while speaking to a group of U.S. bishops:

> The statement of the U.S. bishops' pro-life committee, 'Nutrition and Hydration: Moral and Pastoral Considerations,' rightly emphasizes that the omission of nutrition and hydration intended to cause a patient's death must be rejected and that, while giving careful consideration to all the factors involved, the presumption should be in favor of providing medically assisted nutrition and hydration to all patients who need them.[3]

"Spiritual Purpose" Rationale

The Holy Father's new speech is more forthright than past U.S. bishops' statements in identifying assisted feeding as part of the "normal care due to the sick" even in cases where specific medical treatments have been withdrawn. On this point, however, there is precedent in documents issued by several Vatican advisory bodies in recent years, including the Pontifical Council *Cor Unum* and the Pontifical Council for Pastoral Assistance to Health Care Workers. In 1995, for example, the latter body's *Charter for Health Care Workers* stated: "The administration of food and liquids, even artificially, is part of the normal treatment always due to the patient when this is not burdensome for him: their undue suspension could be real and properly so-called euthanasia" (n. 120).

Late in 2002, a leading proponent of the "spiritual purpose" rationale for withdrawing assisted feeding from patients in a vegetative state expressed concern over recent statements by Church officials and Vatican theologians on life support, beginning with certain passages of the Holy Father's 1995 encyclical *Evangelium vitae*. He suggested then that a "development of doctrine" may be taking place, narrowing the circumstances under which assisted feeding and other life support may be withdrawn.[4] Whether one sees this trend as a development of doctrine will depend on one's interpretation of Church teaching prior to 1985; in any case, this account shows that the Pope's new speech is not a radical shift but the culmination of a longstanding trend at the Vatican.

Notably, in the March 20 speech, food and fluids are identified as normal care not only to emphasize the strong presumption in favor of their use but also to counter an argument sometimes used to justify their withdrawal from seemingly incurable patients: The argument that such means should be assessed in terms of whether they lead to recovery from the patient's underlying condition. The Holy Father emphasizes that assisted feeding is not a "medical act" in this sense—that is, it should not be dismissed as useless or "extraordinary" because it preserves life and prevents a death from starvation or dehydration but does nothing more. Life itself is sufficient reason to continue such support.

> The evaluation of probabilities, founded on waning hopes for recovery when the vegetative state is prolonged beyond a year, cannot ethically justify the cessation or interruption of *minimal care* for the patient including nutrition and hydration. (n. 4, original emphasis)

In this commentator's view, the Holy Father has not declared an absolute moral obligation to provide assisted feeding in all cases, regardless of whether it effectively provides nourishment or might in a given case impose grave suffering and other burdens on a patient. But he has established the provision of food and fluids as a general norm for all helpless patients, including those who seem completely unresponsive to the outside world. It is in serving those who may never visibly respond to our care that we find the ultimate test of our Christian charity and our respect for the inherent dignity of each human life.

Notes

1. Congregation for the Doctrine of the Faith, *Declaration on Euthanasia*, part IV.

2. See http://www.usccb.org/prolife/issues/euthanas/nutindex.htm.

3. "Building a Culture of Life," 'ad limina' address to the bishops of California, Nevada, and Hawaii (October 2, 1998), *Origins* 28(18): 4.

4. Kevin O'Rourke, "Ms. 'B' and the Vatican," *National Catholic Bioethics Quarterly* 2(4): 600.

17

Medically Assisted Nutrition and Hydration: A Contribution to the Dialogue

Mark Repenshek

John Paul Slosar

The *Address to Participants in the International Congress on "Life-Sustaining Treatments and the Vegetative State: Scientific Advances and Ethical Dilemmas,"* promulgated in March of this year by Pope John Paul II, has become a source of considerable controversy, partly due to the theological and clinical complexity of this issue, and partly because of how it has been portrayed in the popular media.[1] In light of this controversy, many Catholics, as well as Catholic health systems, are re-examining the half-millennium-old tradition of Catholic moral teaching regarding the obligation to use particular means of sustaining human life.[2] In this essay, we seek to foster that effort. In light of that tradition, and particularly the discussion of the principles of proportionate and disproportionate means, we will propose a way of interpreting the recent papal address that has not received significant attention.

The Duty to Sustain Life

Perhaps the most fundamental tenet of the Roman Catholic moral tradition is that life is a precious gift from God.[3] This conviction is the basis for a duty to protect and preserve our lives, but that duty does not imply an obligation to use every and all means available to sustain our lives at all costs.[4] Catholic moral teaching holds that the ultimate end of human life lies with God and that life on earth is itself only a penultimate good. As Pope Pius XII notes, "Life, health, all temporal activities are in fact subordinated to spiritual ends."[5] Reaffirming this insight, Pope John Paul II wrote in *Evangelium Vitae* that "it is precisely [our] supernatural calling which highlights the *relative character* of each individual's earthly life. After all, life on earth is not an 'ultimate' but a 'penultimate' reality."[6]

Thomas Shannon and James Walter have recently pointed out that the resulting duty to sustain life has traditionally been understood in the Roman Catholic moral tradition as teleological.[7] In the context of the Catholic moral tradition, "teleological" is not synonymous with consequentialist. Rather, as we understand it, the teleological framework found within the Catholic tradition recognizes the moral relevance both of rules of right conduct and of consequences.[8] In other words, the Catholic moral tradition has always recognized some negative obligations of a fundamentally deontological nature, including of course the obligation never to directly intend the destruction of innocent human life. It is our view, however, that these deontological obligations do not preclude the use of the principles of proportionate and disproportionate means as teleological guides for discerning whether discontinuing a particular life-sustaining treatment would constitute the directly intended destruction of innocent human life.

As defined by the *Ethical and Religious Directives for Catholic Health Care Services* (*ERD*), a proportionate means is one that individuals are obligated to use to preserve life insofar as, in the judgment of the patient, the means in question offer a reasonable hope of benefit *and* do not entail excessive burdens.[9] One is not obligated to use any means of sustaining life that, in one's own judgment, either do not offer a reasonable hope of benefit or entail excessive—that is, disproportionate—burdens. The *Catechism of the Catholic Church* affirms this when it says, "Discontinuing medical procedures that are burdensome, dangerous, extraordinary, or disproportionate to the expected outcome can be legitimate; it is the refusal of 'over-zealous' treatment. Here one does not will to cause death; one's inability to impede it is merely accepted."[10] It is important to note here that neither the *ERD* nor the *Catechism* specify which procedures, diagnostics, or therapies constitute proportionate or disproportionate means. In fact, the *ERD* explicitly emphasize that those determinations are to be made "in the judgment of the patient."

The Vatican's 1980 *Declaration on Euthanasia* reaffirms these principles and the nature of the moral obligation to use particular means of sustaining life. It stated: "It will be possible to make a correct judgment as to the means by studying the type of treatment to be used, its degree of complexity or risk, its cost and the possibilities of using it, and comparing these elements with the result that can be expected, taking into account the state of the sick person and his or her physical and moral resources."[11] Likewise, Pope John Paul II wrote in his 1995 encyclical letter *Evangelium Vitae*, "Certainly there is a moral obligation to care for oneself and to allow oneself to be cared for, but this duty must take account of concrete circumstances. It needs to be determined whether the means of treatment available are objectively proportionate to the prospects for improvement."[12]

The meaning of the term "concrete circumstances," although potentially ambiguous, has traditionally been understood to include the effects of treatment upon family members and the community. The *Declaration on Euthanasia* speaks to this point, noting: "This rejection of a remedy is not to be compared to suicide; it is more justly to be regarded as a simple acceptance of the human condition or a desire to avoid the application of medical techniques that are disproportionate to the value of the anticipated results or, finally, a desire not to put a heavy burden on the family or the community."[13]

Origins of the Principles

While recent Church teaching regarding the principles of proportionate and disproportionate means has focused on medical treatments, early attempts to articulate the principles also addressed non-medical means of prolonging life. In the sixteenth century, the Spanish Dominican theologian Francisco de Vitoria (1486–1546) explicitly addressed the issue of what one is obliged to undergo to prolong life in his *Relectiones Theologiae*. Vitoria considered one's obligation to eat certain foods: "If a sick man can take food or nourishment with some hope of life, he is held to take the food, as he would be held to give it to one who is sick. [However], if the depression of spirit is so low and there is present such consternation in the appetitive power that only with the greatest of effort and as though by means of certain torture, can the sick man take food, right away that is reckoned a certain impossibility, and therefore he is excused, at least from mortal sin, especially where there is little hope of life or none at all."[14]

Expanding on this basic conviction, theologians Domingo Bañez (1528–1604) and Spanish Jesuit cardinal John de Lugo (1583–1660) introduced the terms "ordinary" and "extraordinary," which are synonymous with the now more predominant terms "proportionate" and "disproportionate."[15] Each of these authors qualifies and defines the parameters of these terms and applies them to the use of food and other natural means in the preservation of human life. For example, de Lugo considers the example of a religious novice in ill health who is advised to leave the religious community and return to the world in order to seek food and surroundings that would be more conducive to his health, and possibly prolong his life. The question de Lugo explicitly considers is whether the novice is obligated to leave the community for the sake of conserving his life even though doing so would entail significant spiritual sacrifice. Ultimately, de Lugo concludes that the novice is not obligated to leave the community; he is obligated only to use the means available to him within the community. The point, then, is that what constitutes ordinary or proportionate means is not necessarily determined by what is common, nor even by whether the means used are medical or natural, but by their effect on one's status or condition in life, on one's financial, social, physical, spiritual, and psychological condition.[16]

Ultimately, five criteria under which any means of sustaining life could be considered extraordinary or disproportionate emerged from the writings of these theologians. These criteria included any means of sustaining life that either (1) simply could not be obtained because one does not have access to them, (2) could be obtained only with the greatest of effort or involve circumstances of danger or grave inconvenience, (3) entail intense pain, (4) entail excessive costs, or (5) entail intense fear or strong psychological repugnance. It is important to note that these criteria applied even if the means in question offered a certain hope of success. In 1958, Pope Pius XII (1876–1958), in an address to an International Congress of Anesthesiologists, further refined a conception of extraordinary or disproportionate means as comprising all medicines, treatments, and operations that cannot be obtained or used without excessive expense, pain, or other inconvenience, or which, if used, would not offer a reasonable hope of benefit. He wrote, "Normally one is held to use only ordinary means—according to circumstances of persons, places, times, and culture—that is to say, means that do not involve any grave burden for oneself or another. A more strict obligation would be too burdensome for most men and would render the attainment of the higher, more important good too difficult."[17] This articulation of the principles emphasized the role of proportionate reason contained within the five traditional criteria and was reiterated in the *Declaration on Euthanasia*. This understanding has become the predominant lens through which the means of sustaining life are deemed either morally obligatory or optional.

The Papal Address

In recent decades, two extreme views have emerged concerning medically assisted nutrition and hydration for persons in a persistent vegetative state (PVS). One view considers it always obligatory as long as it sustains physiologic life; the other considers it never obligatory insofar as there is only a very small probability that such individuals will ever regain consciousness.[18] As we read the Papal address, we think it is intended to provide a number of clarifications related to these extreme positions.

First, in opposition to some contemporary views that the value of human life is dependent on one's ability to function, the address affirms the intrinsic value and personal dignity of every human person, irrespective of their disability or medical condition, and in particular irrespective of whether they are in a PVS.[19] The address emphasizes that persons in a PVS are among some of the most vulnerable members of society and, as such, calls upon "professional ethics and human and Christian solidarity" to recognize "those patients whose human dignity remains intact though they are unconscious and unable to speak for themselves."[20]

Read in this context, the address seems to focus on the obligations of physicians and health care professionals who might base a decision to withdraw medically assisted nutrition and hydration on *external quality of life* judgments, insofar as the direct intention would be to hasten the death of the patient.[21] If one reads the address as consistent with previous papal teaching regarding the use of life-sustaining means, then it is precisely such decisions, done to directly intend to hasten the death of the patient, that are considered problematic and morally illicit.[22] Understood in this way, the address does not necessarily preclude health care providers from honoring advance directives or appropriate surrogate decisions to refuse medically assisted nutrition and hydration in the case of PVS. Rather, it establishes that because a person in a PVS maintains his or her inherent dignity and worth, external quality of life judgments cannot serve as the *sole* basis for withdrawing medically assisted nutrition and hydration. If this interpretation is right, then we do not read the address as the "significant departure from the Roman Catholic bioethical tradition" that Shannon and Walter have called it.[23] Rather, we view it as one possible application of the principles of proportionate and disproportionate means to a narrowly construed set of circumstances.

Within this application, the address identifies nutrition and hydration, even when delivered via artificial means, as a form of basic care. The implication of these statements is that persons in a PVS have a basic human right to access medically assisted nutrition and hydration along with other forms of basic care, such as cleanliness and warmth. However, given the origins of the principles and given what it means to have a right to something,[24] the address does not imply that medically assisted nutrition and hydration is obligatory for all patients in a PVS. As noted in the address itself, such care is only "*in principle*, ordinary and proportionate, and *as such* morally obligatory, insofar as and until it is seen to have attained its proper finality, which in the present case consists in providing nourishment to the patient and alleviation of his suffering" (emphasis added).[25] But even though medically assisted nutrition and hydration should be considered in principle ordinary and proportionate, the address does not state that an individual could not judge *for themselves* that medically assisted nutrition and hydration in the case of PVS would be disproportionate means in the actual circumstances of his or her own life. Nor does "*in principle*, ordinary and proportionate, and as such morally obligatory," imply that such a judgment would not be permissible. Rather, the implication is twofold: (1) that it would not be morally appropriate to consider medically assisted nutrition and hydration as always and everywhere disproportionate simply because a person is in a PVS; and (2) that a particular individual is not required to consider medically assisted nutrition and hydration always and everywhere ordinary and proportionate, independently of any considerations regarding his or her own *circumstances*. As we understand it, then, "in principle ordinary and proportionate" does not mean "without exception," but only "all other things being equal."

In this way, the address seems to be affirming the "presumption in favor of providing nutrition and hydration to all patients" that is already found in directive fifty-eight of the ERDs: "There should be a presumption in favor of providing nutrition and hydration to all patients, including patients who require medically assisted nutrition and hydration, *as long as* this is of sufficient benefit to outweigh the burdens involved to the patient" (emphasis added). In other words, withdrawal of medically assisted nutrition and hydration should not be viewed as *automatically indicated* for the entire class of PVS patients because of external judgments that their quality of life is so low that medically assisted nutrition and hydration is of absolutely no benefit.

In short, if the address is interpreted in light of previous papal teaching and the broader Catholic moral tradition, as we believe it should be, then its consequences would not be as dire as those that Shannon and Walter describe. The address holds quite simply that medically assisted nutrition and hydration for PVS cannot always and everywhere be considered either proportionate or disproportionate; instead, its status depends on the circumstances of individual cases. Of course, the full practical implications of the address depend largely on how Catholic bishops receive and interpret it. This essay has been intended only as a contribution to the ongoing reflection and dialogue that must accompany any interpretation of the address and as such is open to later revision and qualification.

Notes

1. The text of this address is from the English translation found on the Vatican website: http://www.vatican.va/holy_father/john_paul_ii/speeches/2004/march/documents/hf _jp-ii_spe_20040320_congressfiamc_en.html.

2. See D. O'Brien, J. P. Slosar, and A. R. Tersigni, "Utilitarian Pessimism, Human Dignity, and the Vegetative State," *The National Catholic Bioethics Quarterly* 4 (3): 497–512; T. A. Shannon and J. J. Walter, "Artificial Nutrition, Hydration: Assessing Papal Statement," *National Catholic Reporter,* April 16, 2004, at http://natcath.org/NCR_Online/archives2/2004b/041604/041604i .php; R. Hamel and M. Panicola, "Must We Preserve Life?" *America* 190 (April 19, 2004): 6–8; G. D. Coleman, "Take and Eat: Morality and Medically Assisted Feeding," *America* 190 (April 5, 2004); and P. J. Cataldo, "Pope John Paul II on Nutrition and Hydration: A Change of Catholic Teaching?" *The National Catholic Bioethics Quarterly* 4 (3): 513–36.

3. Pope John Paul II, *"Evangelium Vitae"* (March 25, 1995), *Origins* 24 (42), n. 2.

4. M. Panicola, "Catholic Teaching on Prolonging Life: Setting the Record Straight," *Hastings Center Report* 31 (6): 18, 21–22; Hamel and Panicola, "Must We Preserve Life?," 7; T. R. Kopfensteiner, "Developing Directive 58: A Look at the History of the Directive on Nutrition and Hydration," *Health Progress* 81 (3): 21; T. A. Shannon and J. J. Walter, "The PVS Patient and the Foregoing/Withdrawing of Medical Nutrition and Hydration," *Theological Studies* 49 (4): 633–34, 644–45; B. M. Ashley and K. O'Rourke, *Health Care Ethics: A Theological Analysis,* fourth edition (Washington, D.C.: Georgetown University Press, 1997), 425; and R. A. McCormick, "To Save or Let Die: The Dilemma of Modern Medicine" and "The Moral Right to Privacy," both in *How Brave a New World? Dilemmas in Bioethics* (Washington, D.C.: Georgetown University Press, 1981), 345–48 and 367–68 respectively.

5. Pope Pius XII, "The Prolongation of Life," (November 24, 1957), *Pope Speaks* 4 (4): 395–96.

6. Pope John Paul II, *"Evangelium Vitae,"* Introduction, Section 2.

7. T. A. Shannon and J. J. Walter, "Implications of the Papal Allocution on Feeding Tubes," *Hastings Center Report* 34 (4): 18–20.

8. P. Knauer, "The Hermeneutic Function of the Principle of Double Effect," in *Readings in Moral Theology: Moral Norms and the Catholic Tradition,* ed. C. E. Curran and R. A. McCormick (New York: Paulist Press, 1979), 1–39; R. A. McCormick, "Ambiguity in Moral Choice," in *Doing Evil to Achieve Good: Moral Choice in Conflict Situations,* ed. R. A. McCormick and P. Ramsey (Chicago, Ill.:

Loyola University Press, 1978), 7–53; L. Janssens, "Ontic Evil and Moral Evil," *Louvain Studies* 4 (1972): 115–56; T. O'Connell, *Principles for a Catholic Morality* (San Francisco, Calif.: HarperSan-Francisco, 1990).

9. United States Conference of Catholic Bishops, *Ethical and Religious Directives for Catholic Health Care Services*, fourth edition (Washington D.C.: United States Catholic Conference, 2001), nos. 56 and 57.

10. *Catechism of the Catholic Church* (Washington, D.C.: United States Catholic Conference, 1994), no. 2278.

11. Congregation for the Doctrine of the Faith, "Declaration on Euthanasia," section 4, found at: http://www.vatican.va/roman_curia/congregations/cfaith/documents/rc_con _cfaith_doc_19800505_euthanasia_en.html.

12. Pope John Paul II, *"Evangelium Vitae,"* no. 65.

13. Congregation for the Doctrine of the Faith, "Declaration on Euthanasia," section 4.

14. F. de Vitoria, *On Temperance in Reflection on Homicide and Commentary on* Summa Theologiae II–II q. 64 (Thomas Aquinas), trans. John P. Doyle (Milwaukee, Wis.: Marquette University Press, 1997).

15. Panicola, "Catholic Teaching on Prolonging Life," 15–17.

16. D. A. Cronin, "Conserving Human Life: Part I," in *Conserving Human Life*, ed. R. E. Smith (Braintree, Mass.: The Pope John Center, 1989).

17. Pope Pius XII, "Address to an International Congress of Anesthesiologists," sub-heading, "Basic Principles," found at: http://lifeissues.net/writers/doc/doc_31resuscitation .html.

18. For examples of the extreme views concerning obligations toward PVS patients, see W. E. May et al., "Feeding and Hydrating the Permanently Unconscious and Other Vulnerable Persons," in *Quality of Life: The New Medical Dilemma*, ed. J. J. Walter and T. A. Shannon (New York: Paulist Press, 1990), 195–202; and P. Singer, *Rethinking Life and Death: The Collapse of Our Traditional Ethics* (New York: St. Martin's Press, 1994), 70–75. An extensive medical literature addresses the probability of recovering consciousness; for a good introduction, see Multi-Society Task Force on PVS, "Medical Aspects of the Persistent Vegetative State," *NEJM* 330 (1994): 1499–1508, 1572–79.

19. Pope John Paul II, "Life-Sustaining Treatment and Vegetative State: Scientific Advances and Ethical Dilemmas," no 3.

20. Ibid., no 4.

21. Ibid., no 5.

22. Ibid., no 4.

23. Shannon and Walter, "Implications of the Papal Allocution on Feeding Tubes," 18.

24. Regarding our understanding of what it means to say that someone has a right to something, see O'Brien, Slosar, and Tersigni, "Utilitarian Pessimism, Human Dignity, and the Vegetative State," 502–8.

25. Pope John Paul II, "Life-Sustaining Treatment and Vegetative State: Scientific Advances and Ethical Dilemmas," no 4.

18

Assisted Nutrition and Hydration and the Catholic Tradition

Thomas A. Shannon

James J. Walter

The Terri Schiavo case in Florida focused attention on a variety of issues related to the end of life: who is the decision maker, the status of advanced directives, the role of family members with respect to married adult children, and issues related to the removal of life support systems, particularly assisted nutrition and hydration. Terri Schiavo is now linked to two other young women who played a critical role in helping us to think through ethical issues at the end of life. Karen Ann Quinlan and her family raised the issue of the removal of a ventilator. In her case the physicians were reluctant to do this because they feared legal repercussions. The legal and ethical analysis concurred that such removal was justified because it constituted extraordinary means of treatment. Nancy Cruzan and her family focused attention on the removal of artificial nutrition and hydration (ANH). Again law and ethics concurred that such removal was justified, particularly because people testified that being maintained in such circumstances were not her wishes.

On February 25, 1990, Terri Schiavo had suffered a heart attack, possibly brought on as a result of chemical imbalances from an eating disorder. She suffered loss of oxygen to her brain and was eventually diagnosed as being in a persistent vegetative state. A decade later, in February 2000, her husband Michael Schiavo requested that her feeding tube be removed. The Circuit Court judge agreed, and this set off a lengthy appeal and counter-appeal process, including attempted legislative initiatives from the state of Florida and the United States Congress and thirty-seven court reviews, that were complicated by increasing family acrimony and public commentary from a variety of sources: religious, political, ethical, and legal. After a five-year legal battle, the feeding tube was removed, and Terri Schiavo died on March 31, 2005, at the age of forty-one.

A critical element in the debate was the ethics of the use of feeding tubes for patients in a persistent vegetative state. Several bishops, particularly in light of the papal allocation on feeding tubes in March 2004, argued that their use was morally obligatory. Thus Bishop Vaga of Baker, Oregon: "She may well die in the future from an inability to digest food but it would be murder to cause her death by denying her the food she still has the ability to digest and which continues to provide for her a definite benefit—life itself."[1] That sentiment was echoed by Representative Thomas DeLay of Texas who said: "That act of barbarism can be and must be prevented."[2] A comment on the ethical issue underlying the provision of ANH was offered by Bishop Loverde of Arlington, Virginia, who said: "If Mrs. Schiavo were facing imminent death, or were unable to receive food and water without harm, then removing nutrition and hydration would be morally permissible. It is however never permissible to remove food and water to *cause* death. Food and water are basic human needs, and therefore basic human rights."[3] And Richard Doerflinger of the United States Catholic Conference of Bishops was reported to have articulated the normative nature of this position in an interview with the *Washington Post*:

Before the pope made his statement about feeding-tube cases at a conference last year there was enough uncertainty about the church's position that Catholics could remove feeding tubes without fear of committing a sin. No one could fairly have said to you that you were dissenting from clear Catholic teaching. Now you would have to say, "Yes, you are."[4]

The issue on which we focus in this note is the state of the question in the Catholic tradition regarding the use of assisted nutrition and hydration, an issue that became central in the media and in public debate.

Our position is that there have been four unacknowledged shifts within the last twenty-five years from the traditional method of analyzing our moral obligations during illness and the dying process. The first of these is a shift in the very method itself: from proportionate reasoning as in the "Declaration on Euthanasia" from the Congregation for the Doctrine of the Faith in 1980 to a deontological reasoning as in the March 2004 papal allocution "Care for Patients in a 'Permanent' Vegetative State." Second, there is a shift in applying the ordinary–extraordinary distinction from the general context of obligations to oneself while ill to restricting the application to the context of imminent dying. Third, there has been a shift from making a determination of whether or not to use an intervention such as chemotherapy or assisted nutrition and hydration to a presumption in favor of using such interventions. Finally, following John Paul II's allocution, there is a shift from a presumption to use to an obligation to use. Thus, in a series of statements from various ecclesial commissions and magisterial authorities, the tradition has been moved recently from both a patient-centered focus and obligations determined through the use of proportionate reason to a technology and intervention-centered focus with obligations being determined by deontological principles. We call this more recent position the revisionist position.

The Development of the Revisionist Position

Methodological Shift

Many moral theologians argue that there are two different ethical methodologies operating in Roman Catholicism. The first is deontological or a principle-based ethic and is used primarily in the areas of sexual morality and in medical morality where sexual morality is the content, e.g., assisted reproduction. The resolutions of ethical issues are deducted from the principles and there are no exceptions to the principles and no parity of matter in sexual issues. The principles bind absolutely and are not qualified by circumstances. The other method is the one used in the area of social justice, for example in the analysis of the morality of war or economic policy. This method, used in the two pastoral letters of the United States bishops *The Challenge of Peace* in 1983 and *Economic Justice for All* in 1986, includes scriptural and philosophical perspectives, empirical analysis, expert testimony, and an examination of a variety of contexts and circumstances. The conclusions drawn are recognized to be provisional in that new data can reshape the conclusion, and there is a recognition that one can come to different conclusions that are in harmony with one's starting principles.

Historically, the method of analysis of issues related to end-of-life issues has mostly utilized the second method. This ethic has traditionally been patient-centered and focused on an evaluation of benefits and burdens or on whether the intervention was proportionate or disproportionate. This is the method of, for example, the 1980 "Declaration on Euthanasia" from the Congregation for the Doctrine of the Faith.

First the Congregation notes that it "pertains to the conscience either of the sick person, or of those qualified to speak in the sick person's name, or of the doctors, to decide, in the light of moral obligation and of the various aspects of the case" (IV). The "Declaration" says that the patient can make a correct decision about whether a treatment is proportionate or disproportionate by "studying the type of treatment to be used, its degree of complexity or risk, its cost and the possibilities of using it, and comparing these elements with the result that can be expected, taking into account the state of the sick person and his or her physical and moral resources." (IV). Finally, the "Declaration" notes that one can refuse treatments based on a "desire not to impose excessive expense on the family or the community" (IV).

This position is essentially supported by the Pontifical Council Cor Unum when it says:

> The fundamental point is that the decision should be made according to rational arguments that have taken well into account the many and various aspects of the situation, including what effect will be had upon the family. The principle to follow is, therefore, that no moral obligation to have recourse to extraordinary measures exists; and that, incidentally, a doctor must follow the wishes of a sick person who refuses such measures.[5]

The "Declaration on Euthanasia" is a clear and articulate summary of the moral teaching of the Catholic Church on end-of-life issues from about the sixteenth century to the present. Many of these teaching are summarized in the doctoral dissertation by now Bishop Daniel Cronin.[6] The constant theme of the moralists is that the patient needs to determine what is extraordinary in light of his or her medical circumstances, financial situation, and values. If the effects of the intervention are disproportionate to the desired outcome, they need not be used.

However, a shift seems to be occurring in this tradition and in the method over the past two and half decades. When one reads the 2004 allocution by John Paul II on assisted nutrition and hydration, there is a methodological shift to deontology and determination of principles by definition or stipulation. Briefly, the pope stated that such tubes were "not a medical act" and their use "always represents a natural means of preserving life" and is part of "normal care." Therefore, their use is to be considered in principle ordinary and obligatory. "If done knowingly and willingly" the removal of such feeding tubes is "euthanasia by omission." The person's medical condition is not really relevant in making a determination about the use of feeding tubes, except if the body cannot assimilate the fluids or the intervention does not alleviate the suffering of the patient, because the food and water delivered through such tubes is ordinary care and provides a benefit—"nourishment to the patient and alleviation of his suffering."[7]

What is interesting about this papal allocution is that it seems to represent a significant departure from the Roman Catholic bioethical tradition with respect to both the method and the basis upon which such decisions are made. Historically, the method for making a determination about the use of a medical intervention was the proportion between the benefits of the intervention and its harms or burdens to the individual, family, and community. The method is a teleological balancing of the impact of the intervention. This has been the central teaching of the tradition from the mid-1600s through Pope Pius XII and the 1980 "Declaration on Euthanasia" by the Congregation for the Doctrine of the Faith.[8] The method announced by Pope John Paul II appears to be deontological in nature. The use of feeding tubes to deliver artificial nutrition and hydration is stipulated as in principle ordinary, and such an intervention apparently must not be forgone or withdrawn unless or until the body cannot assimilate the nutrients or they do not alleviate the suffering of the patient.[9]

The Shift from Illness to Imminent Dying

When one reads the manualist tradition on this question, the general framing of the question is in terms of preserving one's life during an illness. Historically, particularly up to about 1950, there was a coincidence of becoming ill and dying but that was because of the general lack of any genuinely useful medical interventions. Typically when one got seriously ill, one died. However, the moralists did not cast the teaching as applicable only in the context of dying. For example, when Francisco de Vitoria in the sixteenth century spoke of "protecting his life," of "employing all the means to conserve his life," he believed that "one is not held to lengthen his life."[10] Thomas Sanchez, in the same century, says that, "it is inferred that one is not obliged to use medicines to prolong life even where there would be the probable danger of death, such as taking a drug for many years to avoid fevers."[11] Thus the obligation is cast in terms of the general context of illness and the prolongation of life.

Pius XII, in his 1957 address on "The Prolongation of Life," discusses the possibility of terminating attempts at resuscitation by not placing a patient on a mechanical ventilator. In this address the discussion of termination of life support occurs within the context of deep unconsciousness and hopelessness but not within the context of dying or of terminal illness. Additionally, Pius does not posit a presumption to resuscitate but rather uses the traditional burden–benefit method to determine whether there is an obligation to resuscitate.[12]

Finally, the "Declaration on Euthanasia" speaks in this vein as well. Section IV, as noted earlier, discusses the issue under the rubric of caring for one's health and how to determine what remedies to use. The last six sentences of section IV refer to the dying process but only in that one can refuse "means of treatment that would only secure a precarious and burdensome prolongation of life. . . ." (IV). The condition of dying or being terminally ill is not the general context for the application of the decision making process but rather one more situation in which one can apply the method of analysis.

A shift in analysis seems to stem from *Evangelium vitae* in which John Paul II, in talking about aggressive medical therapies that are disproportionate or too burdensome, says "in such situations, when death is clearly imminent and inevitable, one can in conscience" (65) refuse treatments. The footnote for this section is to the CDF "Declaration on Euthanasia," but this seems to misrepresent what the document says. The "Declaration" does talk about imminent death in section IV, but it does not do it in the manner that *Evangelium vitae* suggests. *Evangelium vitae* restricts the application of the criteria of proportionality and burden to the situation of imminent and inevitable death. But this is not what the CDF document says. Rather the analysis of section IV is to identify the method of decision making and what is to be included in it as the patient makes decisions about his or her treatment. The context of dying is yet another time when this method can be brought to bear on the situations. The restriction of the application of the ordinary–extraordinary distinction to imminent death is new and has not been part of the general moral tradition nor of the CDF document.

From the Appropriateness of a Therapy to the Presumption of Its Use

Imbedded in the distinction between ordinary and extraordinary means of medical technology is the possibility of an equivocation on the term "ordinary."

When we discuss medical interventions, we frequently discuss some of them as routine, standard, the treatment of choice, standard of care, or ordinary. What is meant in this discussion is that for this particular situation, this is what is usually or ordinarily done. Such interventions can range from a blood transfusion, to chemotherapy, to cardiac bypass surgery, to dialysis, to the insertion of a feeding tube, etc. However, no determination has yet been made on the effect of such an intervention on the patient or on others. From the perspective of the tradition, this is where the moral evaluation begins. What is the impact on the patient, what benefits or burdens will it bring the patient, what is the likely outcome of the intervention, and what is the cost—both psychological and economic—for the patient and his or her family? The patient must determine whether there is a proportion between what is done ordinarily in medicine and the expected benefits, both short term and long term. What may be *medically* ordinary or routine may not in fact be *morally* ordinary because of a disproportion of the benefit–burden ratio for the patient. We must avoid the common equivocation on the word ordinary.

Another version of this equivocation concerns the distinction as a means of categorizing interventions. When one categorizes medical interventions in the abstract apart from the concrete circumstances of the patient, the basis of the classification itself determines the moral status of the intervention, not the effects of the intervention on the patient. Thus we look at the intervention and ask if this is routinely done. If the answer is yes, then we must use it. Again the assumption is that because an intervention is customarily used, it must be morally obligatory. And again the moral analysis is short-circuited because of the equivocation, and one attempts to draw an "ought" or moral obligation directly from an "is" or what is routinely done.

Another problem this equivocation sets up is that the terms ordinary and extraordinary are used as methods of classification or categorizations of interventions. If an intervention is categorized as ordinary—based on the observation that this is customary or ordinary medical practice—then it is morally obligatory. Fortunately, the tradition does not use the terms ordinary and extraordinary as a means of abstract classification but as the conclusion of an argument about the proportion or disproportion of benefits and burdens, as the CDF phrases it. This point was also nicely made by the founder of American Catholic bioethics, Gerald Kelly, SJ, who noted in 1950 that sometimes even "ordinary artificial means are not obligatory when relatively useless."[13] This conclusion led him to revise the definitions of the terms even more carefully, away from any sense of using them as means to categorize the intervention in the abstract to an evaluation of the impact on the patient.

The equivocation on the term ordinary and the use of the terms as means of categorizing interventions set the context for the presumption of use of assisted nutrition and hydration. For example, in 1986, the Committee for Pro-Life Activities of the then NCCB noted that food and water are necessities of life. And since they can be provided without risks and burdens associated with more aggressive life-supporting interventions, there should be a presumption in favor of their use. This idea of a presumption in favor of ANH was reiterated by the New Jersey Catholic Conference in 1987 when it argued against the removal of ANH in the case of Nancy Jobes. The New Jersey Bishops noted a positive duty to prolong human life and, since food and water are basic to human life, they should always be provided.[14] This position was repeated in the *Ethical and Religious Directives for Catholic Health Care Services* issued in 1994 by the NCCB/USCC. After repeating the traditional means of determining burden and benefit, the document states:

> There should be a presumption in favor of providing nutrition and hydration to all patients, including patients who require medically assisted nutrition and hydration, as long as this is of sufficient benefit to outweigh the burdens involved to the patient.[15]

What is interesting is the structure of the sentence. The tradition would usually begin with an analysis of whether there is burden or benefit and then determine whether ANH is required or not. The revisionist position begins with a presumption and then moves to disprove the presumption. The problem with this comes from either an equivocation on the term ordinary or from using the term as a method of classification. The position of the long-standing tradition has been to evaluate the proposed intervention and then come to a moral conclusion.

A final difficulty with this shift concerns determining to what we have presumptive or prima facie obligations. In the tradition, one had a presumptive obligation to preserve one's life, not a presumptive obligation to accept or take any particular medical technology, e.g., mechanical ventilators, heart transplants, or assisted nutrition and hydration. In recent statements, however, patients have a presumptive obligation to take artificial nutrition and hydration. This presumptive obligation can be overridden if and when it can be shown from the circumstances, e.g., the body cannot assimilate the nutrients or the patient is imminently dying or they do not alleviate the suffering of the patient, that this obligation is not one's actual moral obligation.

From Presumption of Use to the Necessity of Use of Assisted Nutrition and Hydration

The first note of a shift away from considering the context of the sick person as morally relevant to decision making at any stage of the illness is in the previously cited Cor Unum document of 1981. This document states that:

> There remains the strict obligation to apply under all circumstances those *therapeutic measures* which are called "minimal": that is, those which are normally and customarily used for the maintenance of life (*alimentation*, blood transfusions, injections, etc.). To interrupt these minimal measures would in practice be equivalent to wishing to put an end to the patient's life.[16]

Note here that feeding is defined as a medical intervention and that there is the presumption of benefit of this intervention.

The Pontifical Academy of Sciences in 1985 noted: "If the patient is in a permanent irreversible coma, as far as can be foreseen, treatment is not required, but all *care* should be lavished on him, *including feeding*."[17] Note here that "feeding" is not placed within the category of "medical treatment" but is defined as "care," which indicates that such interventions are not subject to the normal moral criterion of proportionality between benefits and burdens.

This position is repeated in John Paul II's allocution on assisted nutrition and hydration in which the pope stated in March 2004 that such tubes were "not a medical act" and their use "always represents a natural means of preserving life" and is part of "normal care." Therefore, their use is to be morally considered in principle as ordinary and obligatory. "If done knowingly and willingly" the removal of such feeding tubes is "euthanasia by omission." Other than the inability of the body to absorb the nutrients or that the patient is imminently dying or that the patient's suffering cannot be alleviated, the person's medical condition is not relevant in making a determination about the use of feeding tubes because the food and water delivered through such tubes is ordinary care and provides a benefit—"nourishment to the patient and alleviation of his suffering."[18] Such a shift to the requirement that assisted nutrition and hydration must be used essentially takes the decision about this intervention out of the patient-centered approach that has so characterized the historical tradition of the past.

Conclusions

The Terri Schiavo case provides an interesting insight into a major change in the methodology to determine whether an intervention is a benefit or a burden, whether it is proportionate or disproportionate. To our knowledge, no one in any of the discussions has argued that there is no moral obligation to provide cures or care for those who are ill or in medically compromised positions. At issue is how one determines that obligation. Our observation is that the tradition from at least the sixteenth century through Pius XII, the Congregation for the Doctrine of the Faith in 1980, and the vast majority of moral theologians has determined this obligation by having the patient consider the benefits and burdens of the intervention to determine if they were proportionate or disproportionate. The tradition did not start with assumptions about interventions, nor did it categorize interventions.

Since the early- to mid-1980s, though, a revisionist position has been emerging in the statements from the Pope, Pontifical Academies, Commissions, and Committees that radically change the methodology. These statements categorize interventions and stipulate obligations. The method shifts from proportionality of effects on the patient (teleology) to deontology.

The shift seems to be motivated by two moves: one ethical and the other political.

The ethical move seems to emerge out of an eliding of two distinct but related elements that make up a moral judgment. The axiological element, which is concerned with the determination of value, affirms the value or sanctity of life of the patient. This assessment opposes, correctly, efforts to devalue life lived under difficult circumstances or problematic medical conditions, such as permanent coma. Thus the axiological element of the moral judgment in the Catholic tradition opposes any use of the phrase "quality of life" as a shorthand way of arguing that a patient's life is not worth preserving. The second and distinct element, the normative, is a determination of what obligations I have in the concrete to maintaining this *valued* life. This normative element has traditionally been resolved by determining the burden–benefit ratio of the proposed intervention. Failure to make this important and traditional ethical distinction between axiology and normativity leads one to affirm wrongly that the affirmation of the value or sanctity of life of the patient in and of itself imposes normative obligations with respect to medical interventions. In addition to being the fallacy of deriving an "ought" from an "is," the failure also implicitly may signify a form of vitalism that affirms that biological life is the only or most important value. Finally, the failure to make the distinction leads to a form of a "medical indications policy" as the moral criterion that mandates that particular interventions necessarily must follow from the diagnosis.

The political move both incorporates the failure to make the distinction between the axiological and the normative and incorporates this into the rhetoric of the right to life movement. Thus the rhetoric of the right to life movement focuses on the obligation to maintain biological life under virtually any and all conditions and in the more excessive strands of the movement comes close to committing idolatry by making biological life the only value to be considered. This is certainly not the traditional Catholic "sanctity of life" position, and, in fact, it begins to move this rhetoric into materialism in that biological life is the only or most important value under consideration. There is no doubt that recent magisterial attempts to protect the dignity of unconscious patients are important and utterly necessary, but the movement to require the use of technologies that sustain biological life may in fact have the opposite effect on a society that is prone to devaluing life.[19]

In an earlier article we developed the following position, and we continue to argue that it will serve as an appropriate basis on which to make decisions about the morality of the use of assisted nutrition and hydration.

> When a proposed intervention cannot offer the patient any reasonable hope of pursuing life's purposes at all or can offer the patient a condition where the pursuit of life's purposes will be filled with profound frustration or with utter neglect of these purposes because of the energy needed merely to sustain physical life, then any medical intervention (1) can only offer burden to the life treated, (2) is contrary to the best interests of the patient, (3) can cause iatrogenic harm or risk of such harm, and (4) has reached its limit based on medicine's own principal reason for existence, and thus treatment should not be given except to palliate or to comfort.[20]

The more recent revisionist perspective approaches end-of-life judgments by defining and categorizing particular interventions in the abstract as ordinary, and, on the basis of this maneuver, mandating these interventions. This method that appears to have entered magisterial statements by stipulation undercuts the traditional benefit–burden method and risks imposing great hardship on patients and families at a time of great crisis. We can think of no greater burden to impose on people at this time than to have them feel abandoned by the Church when they are in greatest need of its benefits. Bluntly stated, the Catholic tradition on end-of-life issues has never mandated doing useless or inane things to people in the name of morality. We should not start doing this now.

Notes

1. http://www.catholicmediacoalition.org/bishops%20on%20terri.htm#BishopVasa (accessed April 15, 2005).

2. http://www.cnsnews.com/ViewPolitics.asp?Page=%5CPolitics%5Carchive%5C2005 03%5CPOL20050318c.html (accessed April 15, 2005).

3. http://www.catholicmediacoalition.org/bishops%20on%20terri.htm. Emphasis in the original.

4. Manuel Roig-Franzia, "Catholic Stance on Tube-Feeding Is Evolving," *Washington Post*, March 27, 2005.

5. Pontifical Council *Cor Unum*, *Questions of Ethics Regarding the Fatally Ill and the Dying* (Vatican City: Vatican Press, 1981), 8–9.

6. This dissertation is now included as part I of the book *Conserving Human Life* (Braintree, Mass.: The Pope John XXIII Medical-Moral Research and Educational Center, 1989).

7. John Paul II, "Care for Patients in a 'Permanent' Vegetative State." This allocution can be found on the Vatican website: http://www.vatican.va/holy_father/john_paul_ii/speeches/2004/march/documents/hf_jp-ii_spe_20040320_congress-fiamc_en.html (accessed April 13, 2005); also in *Origins* 33 (April 8, 2004): 737 and 739–40.

8. Congregation for the Doctrine of the Faith, "Declaration on Euthanasia," *Origins* 10 (August 14, 1980): 154–57.

9. John Paul II, "Care for Patients in a 'Permanent' Vegetative State," 739. Though the Pope made an "in principled" argument here, some have not carefully articulated this in their remarks about the allocution. For example, see the published interview noted above with Richard Doerflinger in the *Washington Post*, March 27, 2005.

10. Cronin, *Conserving Human Life*, 34–37.

11. *Ibid.* 43.

12. Pius XII, "The Prolongation of Life" (November 24, 1957), *The Pope Speaks* 4 (1958): 395–98.

13. Gerald Kelly, "The Duty of Using Artificial Means of Preserving Life," *Theological Studies* 11 (1950): 220. See also "Notes," *Theological Studies* 12 (1951): 550–56 for the revised definitions of ordinary and extraordinary.

14. New Jersey Catholic Conference, "Providing Food and Fluids to Severely Brain Damaged Patients," *Origins* 16 (January 22, 1987): 582–84.

15. USCC, *Ethical and Religious Directives for Catholic Health Care Services* (Washington: USCC, 1994), Directive # 58. Interestingly, in the latest version of the ERDs (2001), the introduction to Part V, in which directive # 58 is found, states: "These statements agree that hydration and nutrition are not morally obligatory either when they bring no comfort to a person who is immi-

nently dying or when they cannot be assimilated by the person's body." Note here that a proportion between benefit and burden is not the criterion used.

16. Pontifical Council *Cor Unum*, 8–9 (emphases added).

17. The Pontifical Academy of Sciences, "The Artificial Prolongation of Life," *Origins* 15 (December 5, 1985): 415 (emphases added).

18. John Paul II, "Care for Patients in a 'Permanent' Vegetative State," 739.

19. See Thomas A. Shannon and James J. Walter, "Implications of the Papal Allocution on Feeding Tubes," *Hastings Center Report* 34 (July–August 2004): 18–20.

20. Thomas A. Shannon and James J. Walter, "The PVS Patient and the Forgoing/ Withdrawing of Medical Nutrition and Hydration," *Theological Studies* 49 (1988): 645.

19

Reflections on the Papal Allocution Concerning Care for Persistent Vegetative State Patients

Kevin O'Rourke, OP

I. Introduction

Recently, Pope John Paul II issued a statement in regard to the care of persons in the persistent vegetative state (PVS) (2004). The statement was received with dismay by many people inside and outside the Catholic healthcare ministry (see O'Brien, 2004; Shannon and Walter, 2004). In sum, the Holy Father stated that artificial nutrition and hydration (AHN) was not medical care, but rather comfort care, and in principle should be maintained even if there is no hope that the patient will recover from the debilitated condition of PVS. He also maintained that a patient in PVS remains a person in the full sense of the term, something not denied by Catholic theologians, ethicists and caregivers. Finally, the statement indicated that knowingly and willingly removing AHN from PVS patients is passive euthanasia. Clearly, this was not an infallible or definitive statement of Church teaching; rather it was an authentic or reformable statement (see *Code of Cannon Law* c. 751, 753; Gaillardetz, 2003, 94–99). The purpose of this essay is to examine the allocution of the Holy Father in light of Church teaching in regard to "reformable statements" and then to consider the allocution itself, and finally to respond to the allocution. Thus, this presentation has four parts:

1. A Consideration of the Norms for Accepting Magisterial Teaching
2. A Consideration of the Purpose and Contents of the Allocution

3. Positive Reasons for Disagreement with the Allocution
4. Implications of the Allocution for Catholic Health Care

II. A Consideration of the Norms for Accepting Magisterial Teaching

At one time, the phrase *Roma locuta est, causa finite [sic] est* (Rome has spoken, there-fore all contrary opinions are overruled) indicated the proper response for the loyal Catholic theologians. But in 1990, realizing that many times the Holy See has spoken and later reversed its teaching, the Congregation for Defense of the Faith (CDF) issued a statement in regard to the acceptance of Church teaching, often called *Donum Veritatis* (1990).[1] This document explained the responsibili-ties of theologians and the magisterium of the Church, showing how the two forms of teaching ministry within the Church should work together. The docu-ment outlined four different forms of magisterial teaching. They are:

1. "When the magisterium of the Church makes an infallible pronounce-ment and solemnly declares that the teaching is found in revelation, the assent called for is of theological faith." Many examples of this infallible form of teaching are found in the Council of Trent, the First Vatican Council, or in the Declarations of the Immaculate Conception and the Assumption of the Blessed Virgin Mary into Heaven, in an "extraordi-nary" form of teaching. But examples of this form of teaching may also he found in the universal and ordinary teaching authority of the pope and bishops, such as the statements concerning abortion and euthanasia in the encyclical *The Gospel of Life* (Ratzinger, 1998).

2. "When the magisterium proposes 'in a definitive way' truths concern-ing faith and morals, which even if not divinely revealed are nevertheless strictly and intimately connected with revelation, these must be firmly ac-cepted and held." The statement of Vatican Council I in regard to papal infallibility and truths of the natural law would fit into this category.

3. "When the Magisterium, not intending to act "definitively" teaches a doctrine to aid a better understanding of revelation and makes explicit its content, or to recall how some teaching is in conformity with the truths of faith or finally to guard against ideas that are incompatible with these truths, the response called for is that of religious submission of intellect and will *(obsequium intellectus et voluntatis)*." As then Father, now Cardinal,

Dulles explained, "this third category has long been familiar to Catholics, especially since the popes began to teach regularly through encyclical letters, some two centuries ago. The teaching of Vatican II, which abstained from new doctrinal definitions, falls predominantly within this category" (Dulles, 1991, 694). Truths of this nature are often described as "non-infallible" or reformable or authentic teachings. The teaching of the encyclical *On Human Life* of Paul VI in 1968, in regard to moral means of family limitation, is of this nature.

4. "Finally. . . in order to warn against dangerous opinions which could lead to error, the magisterium can intervene in questions under discussion which involve, in addition to solid principles, certain contingent and conjectural elements. It often becomes possible with the passage of time to distinguish between what is necessary and what is contingent." Cardinal Dulles states that this is a new dimension in Church teaching. As we shall see, the recent allocution of the Holy Father in regard to the care of PVS patients contains certain contingent and conjectural elements. The response to this fourth kind of teaching, referred to in the instruction as prudential teachings, will be our concern.

Response to Prudential Teaching

According to the teaching of *Donum Veritatis*, one's first response to this type of teaching is to accept it with submission of intellect and will *(obsequium intellectus et voluntatis.)* "The willingness to submit to the teaching of the magisterium on matters per se not irreformable must be the rule." But the teaching in question "might not be free from all deficiencies." It might "raise questions regarding timeliness, the form or even the contents of the magisterial intervention." The instruction sets forth several prudential norms for re-examining in humility the argumentation that seems to lead to a conclusion contrary to the magisterial teaching. If after a process of this nature, the theologian for reasons intrinsic to the teaching of the document is not able to give intellectual assent to the teaching, "the theologian has the duty to make known to the magisterial authorities the problems raised by the teaching in itself, in the arguments proposed to justify it or even in the manner in which it is presented." It should be emphasized that the reasons prompting the theologian to withhold assent must be "intrinsic to the teaching" to demonstrate that the reasons in opposition to the magisterial teaching must be historically and theologically accurate, not founded merely upon contrary practice or the difficulty of putting the teaching into practice.

In situations of this nature, the theologian should refrain from giving public expression to the difficulties or discrepancies that are found in the teaching and should not turn to the mass media to confront the teaching of the magisterium. "Respect for the truth as well as for the People of God requires this discretion." Private discussion of the teaching, for example with other theologians or even in scholarly journals would not be prohibited. But clearly unsuitable would be any effort to organize vocal opposition or an appeal to rejection of a magisterial teaching through popular opinion. Some might consider this form of response as contrary to the spirit of honesty and openness that should be part of a theologian's character. However, the common good takes precedence over proving the personal opinion of a theologian, no matter how well founded it might be. Thus, there is a possibility for dissent to prudential teachings of the magisterium described in the instruction of the CDF. But perhaps dissent is too strong a word. It seems a better word might be "disagreement" or even the phrase, "inability to assent for reasons intrinsic to the teaching." Clearly, to describe the response of a loyal theologian to the teaching of the church as dissent might be an exaggeration and also give the impression that the theologian in question is acting in opposition to the Magisterium or has little respect for the role of the Holy Spirit in the life of the church.

A Significant Question

A significant question remains: Does the person who is not a theologian but who has some knowledge of the situation to which the teaching applies have the same rights as the theologians described in the instruction of the CDF? Does a concerned lay person have the same duty as a theologian if he or she perceives from evidence intrinsic to the matter in question that the teaching "might not be free of all deficiencies in regard to timeliness, the form, or even the content of the magisterial intervention." For example, the teaching in question might be based upon scientific facts or professional practices concerning which the lay person has intimate knowledge. It seems the "ordinary believer" would be able to withhold assent, and to communicate the reasons for this state of mind to the magisterial authority, provided the person in question would follow the same process outlined in the instruction for the theologian (Gaillardetz, 2003,

121ff). Above all, the inability to assent must he based on well-formulated historical and theological reasons and the forum for discussion should not be the mass media. This would preclude basing one's position simply upon the fact that the teaching is difficult to follow, or that many people are engaged in practices opposed to the teaching, as seemed to be the basis for most of the opposition in regard to the teaching of Pope Paul VI contained in the encyclical *On Human Life.*

Reason for Donum veritatis

Why was the instruction *Donum Veritatis* promulgated? In a press conference introducing the document, Cardinal Ratzinger, the Praeses of the CDF, admitted that several teachings of the church have been reversed over time: for example, the teaching of freedom of conscience in regard to religion, the separation of church and state, and many statements of the Pontifical Biblical Commission (Dulles, 1991). Anyone familiar with the papal documents *Mirari Vos* of Gregory XVI and *The Syllabus of Errors* of Pius IX will understand the need for considering this fourth type of papal teaching (Chadwick, 1998, 23–25, 168–81). Does the recent statement of Pope John Paul II concerning the care of PVS patients fall into the category of statements that might in time he reversed? The main part of this essay will investigate this question; we shall be concerned with an examination of the "contingent and conjectural statements" of the papal allocution and the suppositions or assumptions upon which they are based. But before proceeding to these considerations, there are two pre-notes which will facilitate our considerations.

Two Pre-Notes

First, we must distinguish clearly between vegetative state (VS) and permanent vegetative state (PVS) because the document under study at times seems to consider them as one. The allocution defines vegetative state as a condition in which "the patient shows no evident sign of self-awareness or of awareness of the environment and seems unable to interact with others or to react to specific stimuli." Neurologists would add to this definition the fact that the patient displays sleep-wake cycles; hence, the patients eyes are often open, but unable to track in a meaningful manner. When discussing PVS the allocution indicates that there is no different diagnosis for it but only "a prognostic judgment that recovery is statistically speaking more difficult." In fact, the transition from VS to PVS is based on more than statistics. It is based upon a presumption that the condition of the patient is irreversible, and this presumption is based upon neurological evidence gained from a lengthy observation of the patient. "Like all medical judgments this presumption is based upon probabilities, not absolutes" (Joint Task Force, 1994).

Secondly, the allocution maintains that decisions to remove life support should not be made on the basis of quality of life "because the intrinsic value and personal dignity of every human being does not change no matter what the circumstances of his or her life." Quality of life is an ambiguous term. Sometimes it is used to signify human dignity, as in the allocution, but sometimes it is used to signify the circumstances resulting from an illness or pathology. When determining whether or not to utilize or withhold life support, as Pope Pius XII observed, an evaluation of the "circumstances of persons, places, times, and culture" (1958) is necessary before making a decision to withdraw life support. The statement of the Pontifical Council *Cor Unum*, quoted with approval in the allocution, referred to this analysis of circumstances as judging "the quality of life" (Pontifical Council *Cor Unum*, 1971). Perhaps when discussing the circumstances which are present in the life of a dying person, we should do away with the term "quality of life" and use the term "quality of function," as suggested by Father Thomas O'Donnell, SJ, a noted medical ethicist, in a private letter many years ago. In this sense, all persons have the same quality of life because God's love extends to every human person no matter how debilitated they might be. But all do not have the same quality of function, and it is the quality of function that we evaluate when questions of prolonging life of ourselves or our loved ones must he settled.

III. A Consideration of the Purpose and Content of the Allocution

Before beginning this part of the presentation, realize that the document under consideration is the allocution as issued by the Vatican Press office, not as it has been interpreted by many individuals and agencies.[2] Some of these interpretations have placed accurately the allocution within the tradition of the church teaching in regard to prolonging life, but it is my contention that the allocution as it stands is in need of revision.

The Goals of the Papal Allocution

Three goals may be discerned from the papal allocution and the conference to which it was presented:

1. The church seeks to counteract the trend in our society and culture toward euthanasia and disrespect for human life. The effort to put people to death to end their suffering or to terminate a debilitated existence is demonstrated in law and medicine in the present time. Euthanasia is legal in some countries and states at this time. Pope John Paul II sought to emphasize that life is sacred and to counteract these vicious trends in the encyclical The Gospel of Life, and carried this message throughout the world on his many journeys.
2. The church wishes to speak on behalf of the debilitated and infirm. Above all, the church seeks to counteract the tendency to have other people decide for the weak and infirm the value of their lives. Fear is expressed that the term "vegetative state" will demean the personal dignity of people in this condition. Thus, the intrinsic value of and personal dignity of debilitated persons is affirmed strongly by John Paul II.
3. Finally, the Holy Father wished to stress that no matter how debilitated and bereft of human function, the infirm are still persons, and to be treated as such by medical personnel, families and society.

No one writing from a Catholic perspective disagrees with the need to work diligently for the attainment of these goals. However, the assumptions upon which a strategy to achieve these goals is based seems subject to question. In the following section, I shall consider two of these assumptions and the conjectural and contingent statements based upon them.

Questionable Assumptions and Statements Based upon Them

The instruction of the CDF states that authentic teachings that contain contingent and conjectural statements may he subject to reversal. According to *Webster's Dictionary*, a conjectural statement is one based on incomplete or inconclusive evidence; a contingent statement is likely to he true, but not yet certain; i.e., it is possible but not certain. Insofar as papal statements of a prudential nature are concerned, the conjectural and contingent statements are based upon assumptions. Thus, an assumption is made that a specific proposition or declaration is true and conclusions are drawn from that assumption; these conclusions are conjectural or contingent, that is, they may or may not be true, depending on the truth of the assumption. In time, an assumption may prove to be untrue, and thus the conjectural or contingent statements which follow from it are also untrue. For example, consider two statements contained in the *Syllabus of Errors* referred to above. In section III of the *Syllabus of Errors*, n. 15, the following statement is condemned: "Every man is free to embrace and profess the religion, which guided by the light of natural reason, he shall consider true." In section VI of the same document, n. 55, the following statement is condemned: "The Church ought to be separate from the State, and the State from the Church." These statements were later reversed by the Second Vatican Council. The Council, in the Decree on Religious Freedom, stated, "that the human person has the right to religious freedom . . . this Council further declares that the right to religious freedom is based on the very dignity of the human person as known through the revealed Word of God and by reason itself" (Flannery, 1980, 800n2). The Council also stated, "The political community and the Church are autonomous and independent of each other in their own fields. Both are devoted to the personal vocation of man under different titles" (Flannery, 800n76).

The assumptions upon which the statements in the *Syllabus of Errors* were founded are not stated in the original documents. But a knowledge of church history helps us discern what they were. First, the church had long maintained that it had some kind of power over secular governments. This assumption dates back to the days when Charlemagne was crowned as Holy Roman Emperor by Pope Leo III in 800, and this assumption found full expression in the encyclical *Unum Sanctam* of Boniface VIII in 1302. Moreover, assumptions were present in the nineteenth century, when the aforementioned statements were condemned by the Holy See, that if people were allowed freedom of religion or if church and state were separate entities that people would lose faith in God and the church, and that the state would persecute and seek to destroy the church. These assumptions proved untrue and thus the contingent and conjectural statements based upon them were later proven untrue and were reversed by the church. At the time they were made, these assumptions were questioned by many and the church suffered embarrassment as a result of the discipline based upon these assumptions (Chadwick, 1998, 168–81).

First Assumption of the Allocution

There are assumptions underlying the recent papal allocution that can be called into question, assumptions that also seem to permeate the thinking of the papal advisors who assisted in the formulation of the allocution.[3] These misleading assumptions lead to contingent and conjectural statements which also may be called into question.

The first assumption that seems to be inconsistent with reality is that there is some hope of benefit from prolonging life for a patient in a permanent vegetative state, even if it is unlikely that the patient will recover. This assumption is held by some theologians and philosophers (Grisez, 1993, 524–26; Grisez, 1990; Boyle, 1995; May et al., 1987) but is contrary to the opinion of several medical societies that have considered the care of patients in this condition (Multi-Society Task Force, 1994a, 1994b; British Medical Association, 2001; American Medical Association, 1992; American Academy of Neurology, 1989), to many theologians and ethicists with clinical experience (Paris, 1998; Broduer, 1990; O'Rourke, 1989; Hamel and Panicola, 2004), and to some members of the hierarchy who have offered guidance to families in specific cases (Gelineau, 1987; Kelly, 1998; Illinois Bishops, 2001). The main support for the opinion that life in PVS is an "intrinsic good" and a "great benefit" is the conviction of the theologian Germain Grisez and his followers that human life is an incommensurable good and that those who deny this assertion are professing dualism (O'Rourke, 1989). If human life is an intrinsic good, why does the church teach that life support may be removed if it imposes an excessive burden? Moreover, as my colleague Benedict Ashley observes:

> the human body is human precisely because it is a body made for and used by intelligence. Why should it be dualism to unify the human body by subordinating the goods of the body to the good of the immaterial and contemplative intelligence? (1994, 73)

While it is not a conclusive proof, it is noteworthy that most of the people who maintain that continued existence in a PVS condition is not a "great benefit" have been involved in clinical and pastoral situations. They are not primarily academic persons; they are physicians, ethicists, and pastoral care personnel who help families make prudential decisions in difficult circumstances. They realize that when families make decisions to remove AHN from PVS patients it is not "tantamount to dumping them in the garbage" (Grisez, 1990, 40). Finally, Bryan Jennett relates the opinions of several groups of clinical practitioners and lay people in regard to having life prolonged in PVS, which opinions are contrary to the assumption that prolonging the life of PVS patients is a great benefit (2002, 73–86).[4]

This first assumption, that life in PVS is a great benefit even if recovery is highly unlikely, leads to a series of contingent and conjectural statements that also can he called into question; statements which seem to remove AHN from the traditional evaluation of hope of benefit because it is presumed that continuation of the persistent vegetative state offers hope of benefit to the patient even though recovery is unlikely. Thus, at best the following statements seem out of touch with reality:

1. "The evaluation of probabilities, founded on waning hope for recovery when the vegetative state is prolonged beyond a year, cannot ethically justify the cessation or interruption of minimal care for the patient, including nutrition and hydration" (para IV). In most cases of PVS, moral certitude that the patient will not recover is possible (Multi-Society Task Force, 1994b). This seems to indicate that there is no hope of benefit to the patient if life support is prolonged by means of AHN.

2. "Death by starvation or dehydration is in fact the only possible outcome as a result of their withdrawal. In this sense it ends up becoming, if done knowingly and willingly, true and proper euthanasia by omission" (para IV). The disturbing implication of this statement is that it gives the impression that the moral object of a human act is determined by the physical result of the action. This of course is contrary to the teaching of the church in the encyclical *The Splendor of Truth (Veritatis Splendor)* (John Paul II, 1993, n. 78). The same physical act may have two distinct moral evaluations; e.g., sexual intercourse may be an act of marital love or an act of adultery. The possibility that AHN might ever be withheld or withdrawn is excluded, if the statement in the allocution is taken literally. In this regard, recall the words of the Document issued by the Pro-life Committee of Bishops in the United States, a document in accord with the basic concepts of the papal allocution:

   We should not assume that all or most decisions to withhold or remove life support are attempts to cause death. Sometimes other causes may be at work, for example, the patient is imminently dying, whether a feeding tube is placed or not . . . at other times, although the shortening of the patient's life is one foreseeable result of an omission, the real purpose of the omission was to relieve the patient or the patient's family (Committee on Pro-Life Activities, 1992, 705ff).

3. "Water and food, even when provided by artificial means, always represents a natural means of preserving life, not a medical act. Its use furthermore should he considered in principle ordinary and proportionate and as such morally obligatory insofar as and until it is seen to have attained its proper finality which in the present case consists in providing nourishment to the patient and alleviation of his suffering" (para IV). Even though the papal allocation maintains, in the face of medical and legal opinion to the contrary (Jennet, 2002, 108ff), that AHN is not medical care, insofar as it "preserves life" it must be morally evaluated by the traditional criteria: hope of benefit and degree of burden (O'Rourke, 1989, 194). Moreover, in so far as "finality" is concerned, as we shall see when considering the second assumption, competent medical opinion holds that people in PVS do not experience pain or suffering.

Second Assumption

The second assumption is even more disturbing than the first. It might be phrased in the following manner: "The medical facts and findings of several professional societies, study groups, research papers, court findings and decisions, are not to be considered as valid scientific evidence." This attitude is disturbing because the Holy See usually encourages and values scientific research and seeks to refer to it when issuing instructions or allocations. The statement of the World Federation of Catholic Medical Associations (FIAMC), which accompanied the allocution, offers inadequate scientific proof for the medical assertions of the allocution. The above assumption leads to the following statements that are contrary to the findings of several different medical research groups and publications:

1. "There are a high number of diagnostic errors reported in the literature" (para II). There are no citations given in the allocution or the statement of the FIAMC to "the literature" in question. No doubt mistakes in diagnosis are possible, but not if diagnoses are made by board-certified neurologists following the guidelines developed by research groups (Jennett, 2002, chap. 2). It has been known for a long time that people

frequently recover from coma and occasionally from VS, but not from PVS that has been properly diagnosed (Levin et al., 1991). As mentioned in the first pre-note, the conditions of coma, VS, and PVS, should not be confused.

2. "Moreover, not a few of these persons, with appropriate treatment and with specific rehabilitation programs have been able to emerge from the vegetative state. . . . We must neither forget nor underestimate that there are well documented cases of recovery even after many years" (para. II). The supposition that recovery from a prolonged vegetative condition or from PVS is likely is also inferred in other parts of the allocution. But on the contrary research publications offer little hope of recovery for PVS patients (Jennett, 2002, chap. 5).

3. "Moreover, it is not possible to rule out a priori that the withdrawal of nutrition and hydration, as reported by authoritative studies is the source of considerable suffering for the sick person, even if we can see only the reaction of the autonomic nervous system or of gestures." Once again, "the authoritative studies" are not cited in the FIAMC statement. Several contemporary studies maintain that removing AHN from patients in PVS or prolonged coma does not cause pain. In the words of one significant study, "The perception of pain and suffering are conscious experiences: unconsciousness by definition precludes these experiences (Jennett, 2002, 15, 17–18; Multi-Society Task Force, 1994b, 1579). With this in mind, describing the removal of AHN as "starving the patient" is a clear misconception.

IV. Positive Reasons for Disagreement with the Allocution

The positive reasons for disagreement with the teaching contained in the allocution are founded upon a Thomistic anthropology of the human person. Briefly, the goal or purpose of human life is friendship with God; i.e., charity (Catechism of the Catholic Church, 1997, n. I; Aquinas, 1966, ST II–II, on charity). To strive for this goal, we must perform human acts. St. Thomas distinguishes between human acts *(actus humanus)* and acts of man *(actus hominis)* (1966, ST I–II, q. I, a. I). Human acts are acts of the intellect and will; acts of man are bodily acts not under the control of the intellect and will, for example, the physiological acts of the body which are not subject to rational activity, such as circulation of blood and digestion. If a person does not have the ability nor the potency to perform human acts now or in the future, then that person can no longer strive for the purpose of human life and it does not benefit the person in this condition to have life prolonged. As Pope John Paul II states in the allocution, "The loving gaze of the Father continues to fall upon them as sons and daughters" but this does not imply that persons in this condition are able to fulfill their part in the reciprocal relationship of friendship, i.e., they are unable to strive for the purpose of life. Therefore, it seems that there is no moral obligation to prolong the life of persons in vegetative states from which they most likely will not recover. Benedict Ashley and I describe the ability to perform a human act as the capacity now, or in the future, to perform acts of cognitive–affective function. If it is morally certain[5] that persons cannot and will not perform acts of this nature now or in the future, then the moral imperative to prolong their lives no longer is present. Hence, it is not a "a great benefit" for the patient, for the family nor for society, to prolong their lives. Moreover, healthcare seeks to help people strive for the purpose of life, not merely to function at the biological level (Pellegrino and Thomasma, 1988, p. 80). Though the sanctity of human life must be affirmed, the fact that death is the gateway to eternal life is often forgotten in contemporary times.

Repetition Lacking

Finally, as of March 30, 2006, the statement of March 20, 2004, has not been repeated by the Holy See. Repetition of an authentic statement is one means that theologians are instructed to use as they evaluate papal teaching. They are told "to assess the nature of the document and the insistence with which a teaching is repeated." (CDF n. 24) (Recall, the March 20, 2004, statement was contained in a papal allocution, the least authoritative form of papal teaching.) If Pope John Paul II wished to repeat the teaching of March 20, 2004, he had a perfect opportunity when he spoke to a conference of health care personnel, *On Palliative Care,* on November 12, 2004. If the teaching was to be interpreted as authentic teaching, this would have been the time to repeat it. Instead, he repeated the traditional teaching in regard to removing life support:

> True compassion encourages every reasonable effort for patient recovery. At the same time, it helps to draw the line when it is clear no further treatment will serve the purpose. . . . Indeed, the object of the decision on whether to begin or to continue a treatment has nothing to do with the value of the patient's life, but rather with whether such medical intervention is beneficial for the patient . . .

the possible decision not to start or to start a treatment will be deemed ethically correct if the treatment is ineffective or obviously disproportionate to the aims of sustaining life or recovering health (John Paul II, 2005, 153–55).

Finally, this opinion is based upon the firm conviction that human life is not an absolute good and that there is life after death, when as the liturgy of the Mass for the Dead explains: "Life is changed, not ended." Thus allowing a person to die when continuing efforts to prolong life offers no hope of benefit or imposes an excessive burden is simply surrendering to God's providence; it is not an act of abandonment.

V. Implications of the Allocution for Catholic Health Care

This section will merely mention some of the difficulties to which this statement gives rise in order to show the ambiguities of the assumptions and the statements based upon them.

1. Advance directives enable people to express their wishes regarding life support if they are unable to speak for themselves as death approaches. If these documents reject the application of AHN if one is in a PVS condition, are they to be followed, or would withdrawal of AHN amount to passive euthanasia? Are these legal documents, which have been approved by many Catholic state conferences in the United States, no longer morally acceptable?

2. The allocution seems to imply that financial considerations are not a factor in making prudential decisions about prolonging life. "First of all, no evaluation of costs can outweigh the value of the fundamental good which we are trying to protect, that of human life." And again the questionable statement: "The care of these patients is not in general particularly costly" (see the allocution para. V). Is this in accord with the tradition of the Church in regard to caring for persons with fatal pathologies?

3. Will Catholic hospitals be required to ensure that all patients, families, and physicians have AHN utilized for all patients in vegetative states or PVS, even if the people in question are opposed to this form of life support?

VI. Conclusion

A fair question would be: What strategy would be useful to attain the goals mentioned earlier in this article? The following actions would seem to contribute to a viable strategy. First, killing of patients, even to alleviate suffering, should be denounced. Second, it seems reliance on the traditional and venerable norms for deciding whether or not to use life support, "hope of benefit" and "degree of burden," should be stressed. Third, guidelines for making decisions concerning hope of benefit and excessive burden should he offered but it should be made clear that these decisions are the responsibility of patients and their proxies, designated either by legal document or custom, and that prudential decisions may differ one person to another. Among these guidelines should be the statement that in itself, prolonging life for patients in PVS or in a state of prolonged coma is not *ipso facto* a "great good" for the patient.

It seems that the present Directive 58 of the *Ethical and Religious Directives (ERD)* of the bishops of the United States concerning this type of decision is adequate, but it could be enhanced by making it more in accord with the terminology of directives 56 and 57. Thus, it seems the Directive 58 should read: "There should be a presumption in favor of providing nutrition and hydration to all patients, including patients who require medically assisted nutrition and hydration. But this presumption gives way if the patient beforehand, or the proxy for unconscious patients, determines that AHN offers no hope of benefit or imposes an excessive burden."

Notes

1. "Instruction on the Ecclesial Vocation of the Theologian." Unless indicated otherwise, all quotations in the text are from this document.

2. For various interpretations see, for example, "Statement of the National Catholic Bioethics Center," April 23, 2004; "Feeding Debate," *Catholic News Service*, April 7, 2004; John Teavis interviews Bishop Sgreccia, and Fathers Mauritio Faggioni, and Brian Johnstone; Richard Doerflinger, *America*, May 3, 2004; Statement of Rev. Dr. Norman Ford, SDB, Chisholm Centre for Health Care Ethics, East Melbourne, Australia; Nicolas Tonti-Phillipini, Canadian Catholic Bioethics Conference 6, 2004; P. Cataldo (2004, pp. 513–37); T. Shannon and J. Walter (2004, pp. 18–20).

3. See, for example, Bishop Sgreccia (2004) and Nancy O'Brien (2004).

4. Other research studies could be cited, but this volume was published recently and contains references to all significant prior studies.

5. Moral certainty is not equated with physical certainty. Rather, it is the certainty in human affairs from what happens "most of the time" *(Ut in pluribus)*. CF. *Summa Theologica*, I–II, q. 96, a.1, ad 3.

References

American Academy of Neurology. 1989. "Position Statement on the Management and Care of the Persistent Vegetative State Patient," *Neurology*, 39:125–26.

American Medical Association, Council on Ethical and Judicial Affairs. 1992. "Decisions near the end of life," *JAMA*, 267:2229–33.

Aquinas, T. 1966. *Summa Theologica*, A. Ross, and P. G. Walsh, (Eds.). Blackfriars edition. New York: McGraw-Hill.

Ashley, B. M. 1994. "What Is the End of the Human Person? The Vision of God and Integral Human Fulfillment," in L. Gormally (Ed.), *Moral Truth and Moral Traditions*, Blackrock, IR: Four Courts Press.

Boyle, J. 1995. "A Case for Sometimes Tube Feeding Patients in Persistent Vegetative State," in J. Keown (Ed.), *Euthanasia Examined* (pp. 189–99). New York: Cambridge University Press.

British Medical Association. 2001. *Withholding and Withdrawing Life-Prolonging Medical Treatment* (2nd ed.). London: BMJ Books.

Broduer, D. 1990. "The Ethics of Cruzan," *Health Progress*, 71:42–47.

Cataldo, P. 2004. "Pope John Paul II, on Nutrition and Hydration," *National Catholic Bioethics Quarterly*, 4 (4): 513–37.

Catechism of the Catholic Church. (1997). Vatican City: Liberia Editrice Vaticana.

Chadwick, O. 1998. *A History of the Popes, 1830–1914*. Oxford: Oxford University Press.

Committee on Pro-Life Activities. 1992. "Nutrition and Hydration: Moral and Pastoral Reflections," *Origins*, 44:705–12.

Congregation for the Doctrine of Faith. 1990. "Instruction on the Ecclesial Vocation of the Theologian," *Origins*, 20 (8): 117–26.

Dulles, A. 1991. "The Magisterium, Theology, and Dissent," *Origins*, 29 (42): 692–96.

Flannery, A., ed. 1980. *Documents of Vatican II: The Conciliar and Post-Conciliar Documents*. Wilmington, DE: Scholarly Resources.

Gaillardetz, R. 2003. *By What Authority?* Collegeville, MN: Liturgical Press.

Gelineau, Bishop. 1987. "On Removing Nutrition and Water from a Comatose Woman," *Origins*, 17:545–47.

Grisez, G. 1990. "Should Nutrition and Hydration Be Provided to Permanently Comatose and Other Mentally Disabled Patients," *Linacre Quarterly*, 57(2): 30–38.

———. 1993. *Living a Christian Life*, Vol. 2. Quincy, IL: Franciscan Press.

Hamel, R., and M. Panicola. 2004. "Must We Preserve Life?" *America*, 190 (14): 6–13.

Illinois Bishops' Pastoral Letter. 2001. Facing the End of Life. *New World Diocesan Paper*, April 15. Chicago, IL.

Jennet, B. 2002. *The Vegetative State, Medical Facts, Ethical and Legal Dilemmas*. New York: Cambridge University Press.

Joint Task Force. 1994. "Medical aspects of the persistent vegetative state," *New England Journal of Medicine*, 330 (31): 1499–1508.

John Paul II. 1993. "Veritas Splendor," *Origins*, 23 (18): 297–334.

———. 2004. "Care for patients in permanent vegetative state," *Origins*; 33 (43): 737–39.

———. 2005. "Address of John Paul II to the participants of the 19th International Conference of the Pontifical Council for Health Pastoral Care, Friday, November 12, 2004." *National Catholic Bioethics Quarterly*, 5 (1): 153–55.

Kelly, Bishop. 1998. Hugh Finn case. Quoted in Paris, J. J., "Hugh Finn's right to die," *America*, 13 (October 31): 13–15.

Levin, H. S., C. Saydjari, H. M. Eisenberg, M. Foulkes, L. F. Marshall, R. M. Ratt, J. A. Jane, and A. Marmarou. 1991. "Vegetative State after Closed Head Injury," *Archives of Neurology*, 48:580–85.

May, W., R. Barry, O. Griese, G. Grisez, B. Johnstone, T. J. Marzen, J. T. McHugh, G. Meilander, M. Siegler, and W. Smith. 1987. "Feeding and Hydrating the Permanently Unconscious and Other Vulnerable Persons," *Issues in Law and Medicine*, 33:203–17.

Multi-Society Task Force. 1994a. "Medical Aspects of the Persistent Vegetative State, Part I," *New England Journal of Medicine*, 330:1499–1508.

———. 1994b. "Medical Aspects of the Persistent Vegetative State, Part II," *New England Journal of Medicine*, 330:1572–79.

O'Brien, N. 2004. "Some Stunned, Others Affirmed by Papal Comments on Feeding Tubes," *Catholic News Service*, April 8, 2004.

O'Rourke, K. D. 1989. "Should Nutrition and Hydration Be Provided to Permanently Unconscious Persons?" *Issues in Law and Medicine*, 5 (2): 181–96.

Paris, J. J. 1998. "Hugh Finn's Right to Die," *America*, 13 (October 31): 13–15.

Pellegrino, E. D., and D. C. Thomasma. 1988. *For the Patient's Good: The Restoration of Beneficence in Health Care.* New York: Oxford University Press.

Pius XII. 1958. "The Prolongation of life," *The Pope Speaks*, 4 (4): 395–98.

Pontifical Council Cor Unum. 1971. *Questions of Ethics Regarding the Fatally Ill and the Dying.* Vatican City: Vatican City Press.

Ratzinger, Cardinal J. 1998. "Commentary on tuendam fidem," *Origins*, 28 (8): 117–19.

Sgreccia, Bishop. 2004. "Preceding the papal allocution," *Catholic News Service*, March 17.

Shannon, T., and J. Walter. 2004. "Implications of the papal allocution on feeding tubes," *Hastings Center Report*, 34 (4): 18–20.

PART SIX

Legal and Public Policy Perspectives

The debate about forgoing or withdrawing artificial nutrition and hydration is not only theological in nature, it also has public policy dimensions, and the debate has taken place in numerous courts and legislatures across the country. Among the more important legal cases are those concerning Clarence Herbert (*Barber v. Superior Court of Los Angeles County*, 1983), Claire Conroy (*In re Conroy*, 1985), Paul Brophy (*Brophy v. New Eng. Sinai Hosp., Inc.*, 1986), Nancy Jobes (*In re Jobes*, 1987), Marcia Gray (*Gray v. Romeo*, 1988), Mary O'Connor (*In re O'Connor*, 1988), Carol McConnell (*McConnell v. Beverly Enterprises*, 1989), Nancy Cruzan (*Cruzan v. Director*, 1990), and Terri Schiavo (e.g., *In re Guardianship of Schiavo*, 2003; *Bush v. Schiavo*, 2004; *Schiavo ex rel. Schindler v. Schiavo*, 2005). It is interesting that the courts have not agreed in their decisions.

State legislatures have also taken up the matter of forgoing or withdrawing nutrition and hydration. In recent years states have enacted legislation that prohibits the withdrawal of artificial nutrition and hydration from patients in PVS or who are otherwise incompetent unless the individual has expressed wishes to the contrary in his or her advance directive. At the conclusion of 2006, largely in response to the Schiavo case, approximately thirteen state legislatures had bills in various stages of the legislative process that would limit the withdrawal of artificial nutrition and hydration from incompetent patients unless they had previously explicitly expressed their wishes. Hence, not only are church officials, theologians, ethicists, and the courts in disagreement over the forgoing or withdrawing of artificial nutrition and hydration, so also are state legislatures.

The purpose of the current section is to offer examples of theological/ ethical reflection on two important legal cases—Clarence Herbert and Claire Conroy. The cases differ somewhat in that Clarence Herbert suffered a profound anoxic brain injury and was said to be in PVS whereas Claire Conroy was awake but severely demented. In both cases lower-court decisions prohibiting the withdrawal of a feeding tube were overturned by higher courts, though for different reasons. The California Court of Appeals in the Clarence Herbert case found that artificial nutrition and hydration could be considered disproportionate given the patient's "hopeless" condition. In the Conroy case the New Jersey Supreme Court, the same court that decided the Quinlan case, based its decision on the rights of incompetent patients, thereby affirming the existence of the incompetent person's right to determine the course of medical treatment exercised through a proxy decision maker.

Most interesting in these cases, and most important, are the presuppositions underlying the court decisions. These presuppositions relate to the nature of artificial nutrition and hydration, the right of an incompetent patient to refuse treatment, quality-of-life judgments and what is to count as burdens and benefits, and the role of intention—the very same issues at the crux of the theological/ethical debate. The articles by John Connery and Richard McCormick offer differing views on these fundamental assumptions. Unless and until there is greater consensus on these basic elements of the debate, it seems unlikely that there can be a consistent public policy, whether issuing from the courts or from legislatures.

20

The Clarence Herbert Case:
Was Withdrawal of Treatment Justified?

John R. Connery, SJ

Clarence Herbert, age fifty-five, was admitted to the Kaiser Permanente Hospital in Harbor City, California, on Aug. 25, 1981, for routine closure of an ileostomy. In the recovery room after the surgery on August 26 he suffered respiratory collapse, which one doctor believed was caused by cardiac arrest. It is not clear how much time elapsed before respiration was restored artificially through a respirator, but the anoxia resulted in severe brain damage. According to the testimony of the nurses and the medical board, the patient was in severe or deep—perhaps irreversible—coma.

The Wayne County medical examiner testified to the brain damage but said that such damage was consistent with a speculative prognosis that the patient could recover but probably not beyond a vegetative state. A neurologist testified that in his belief the patient had a good chance of recovery. It is not clear what he meant by "recovery." My interpretation is that neither thought that the patient was going to die, but at the same time they did not think that he would recover consciousness.

On August 29 Mrs. Herbert signed a consent form indicating that the family wanted all life-sustaining machines removed. At this point the patient was taken off the respirator. Shortly after, all blood tests and all intravenous (IV) fluids were terminated. Then the nasogastric feeding tube was ordered removed. As of August 31, the patient received no further nutrition, hydration, or medication. He was given other care (e.g., he was turned to avoid bed sores, to keep him comfortable, and to relieve other needs), but no life-sustaining measures were used. The patient died on September 6, twelve days after admission to the hospital and six days after termination of life-sustaining treatment.

The district attorney entered a case against the two attending physicians. The charge was murder by deprivation of medical treatment. After studying the case in a preliminary hearing, the magistrate of the Municipal Court dismissed the complaint alleging murder and conspiracy to commit murder by the doctors. He declared further that there was no evidence of unlawful conduct or of malice aforethought on the part of the physicians. This judgment was overruled, and the case was entered in the California Court of Appeals. This court, which filed its decision on Oct. 12, 1983, confirmed the magistrate's judgment; it found that the "omission to continue treatment under the circumstances, though intentional and with knowledge that the patient would die, was not an unlawful failure to perform a legal duty." We are concerned here only with the moral aspect of the case. Our question is, Can the withdrawal of treatment in this case be morally justified?

The first comment that must be made is that the court accounts are in many places unclear. In fact, the absence of much key information makes it impossible to give any categorical response to the actual case. We can only conjure up possible alternatives in the case and respond to them.

The first question that arises concerns the removal of the respirator. It is not clear why this was done so precipitously. According to the account (Magistrate's Findings), the internist removed the patient from the respirator two days after he had been put on it. The account calls this "an unusual procedure" but indicates that the internist ordered it after consulting with the neurologist. It adds that the prognosis at the time was "not absolutely clear" from the record. The patient was clearly in a coma, which may have been irreversible. The neurologists consulted in the case disagreed about the possibility and extent of recovery in such cases, although the weight of opinion seemed to be against a possible return to consciousness.

The magistrate's findings do not indicate whether it was thought that the patient could survive without the respirator. The account refers to the removal of the respirator as an unusual procedure but does not elucidate further. Yet this is relevant to the first moral issue. If it was thought that the patient would die shortly whether on or off the respirator, it would have been morally permissible to remove the respirator as a useless means. If it was thought that the patient might survive indefinitely on the respirator, removing it would have been wrong unless it was an excessive burden for the patient. Generally speaking, short-term use of a respirator would not be considered a heavy burden and so would be obligatory. But long-term use of a respirator, which would have to become a way of life, could easily be judged too burdensome. A competent patient could legitimately refuse this burden. If the patient were comatose, the decision would have to be made by a proxy, but according to the patient's wishes. Since removing the respirator would be permissible in these circumstances, the question to be decided is whether this was or would be the patient's wish. If it was the patient's wish, removing the respirator would have been legitimate. But if it was against the patient's wish, removing the respirator would have been wrong, even if it was judged a morally optional means.

According to the account, on August 29 Mrs. Herbert signed a consent form that stated that the family wanted all life-sustaining machines removed. Since the respirator was removed only after consent had been obtained, it might be concluded that the requirement just discussed was fulfilled. Mrs. Herbert testified that she and her husband had discussed the desirability of having motor support [*sic*] in cases where there is either brain death or severe brain damage. Her husband did not want to be a Karen Quinlan. What is not clear is what prompted the wife and family to give this consent. According to one of the accounts, Mrs. Herbert stated that she had been told that her husband was "brain dead." That she was under this impression can also be gathered from a comment she made regarding the withdrawal of nutrition—she said that one does not "feed a dead man." Although true, the statement did not apply to her husband's case. Unless death can be identified with a comatose condition (which goes against all acceptable criteria for death), it was perfectly clear that the patient was not even "brain dead." So there was no question of removing life support because the patient was dead. If this was the reason for the consent, it did not apply to what was done; that is, the removal of life support from a patient who was still living. So the consent given would have been morally irrelevant.

As is obvious, the above solution contains a lot of "ifs." Whether all these conditions were verified is impossible, at least for this observer, to judge from the written account. One gets the impression of an action that was taken on the basis of some vague generality about a limit to the obligation to treat. The account contains a pitiful lack of the kind of factual information needed for moral discernment.

Providing Nutrition, Hydration

Whatever may have been the expectations, the patient survived removal from the respirator. But two days later, as already mentioned, the attending physician terminated all blood work and all IV fluids. Shortly after that, another attendant ordered removal of the nasogastric feeding tube. From that time until his death on September 6, Mr. Herbert received no nutrition, hydration, or medicine.

Again the account is unsatisfactory and not at all adequate for moral analysis. The only explanation of the removal of the IV given in the account is Mrs. Herbert's statement, already noted, that one does not "feed a dead man." I have already pointed out that consent to the removal of life supports because the patient is already dead would not be valid here, since Mr. Herbert was still alive.

But even if the wife consented to what was actually done, and this consent expressed the clear wishes of the husband, one would still have to assess the withdrawal of the life supports from a moral standpoint. The fact that a patient, or a proxy according to the clear wishes of the patient, consents to something does not automatically make it moral. So the duty to continue the IV, artificial feeding, and other life supports must still be examined.

Here are the traditional norms for judging this duty: If the patient was clearly terminally ill and death was imminent whether the life support was continued or not, one could judge the feeding useless and legitimately discontinue it. No one is obliged to do what is useless. But if the IV feeding would prolong the patient's life—and hence could not be considered useless—would there be an obligation to continue it? As in the case of the respirator, short-term use of life-support therapies to get the patient through a crisis would clearly be obligatory. But the necessity of long-term use, which would have to become a way of life, could easily make it too burdensome. In that event a conscious patient could legitimately decide to forgo it. If the patient were unconscious, the norm set down for a proxy decision would have to be followed: The judgment and decision would have to be based on the patient's wishes. If these were not known, one would have to make a judgment on the basis of what competent patients in general decide in these or similar circumstances.

Again, this discussion of the case has been "iffy" because of the lack of an adequate account of the case. Whether what was actually done could be considered morally legitimate depends on the fulfillment of the conditions required for omitting treatment. Because too much of the necessary factual data is missing or ambiguous, it is impossible to say whether what was actually done was morally permissible.

I have already alluded to the family's apparent misunderstanding about the patient's death. It is not easy to see how the physicians in the case could tolerate this kind of confusion. Apparently, the communication between the physicians and the patient's wife was poor, or at least poorly grasped. It is hard to see how they could have believed that they had "informed" consent to do what they did. It could be, of course, that the physicians themselves did not have a clear idea of what constitutes death and were willing to identify it with "irreversible coma." If so, one cannot lay the confusion at the door of the patient's family. But since such identification is morally unacceptable, it would not justify withdrawing treatment on the grounds that death had occurred. Whatever the physicians' moral stance, they certainly must have known that there is no legal justification in this country for identifying death with irreversible coma.

Treating "Hopeless" Patients

Another problem in the case centers around the use of the term "hopeless." The principle might be put this way: If a patient's condition is hopeless, treatment is useless and therefore not obligatory. Unfortunately, this norm can be ambiguous. A condition may be hopeless in the sense that the disease is incurable. Since there is no successful way of treating this disease, treatment is useless. But is this really relevant to the duty to prolong life? A patient may live a long time with a hopeless disease. Similarly, a particular means may be useless in curing a disease but useful in prolonging life. The facts that it will not cure the disease and that no cure is known for that disease have nothing to do with the duty to use the means to prolong life. If it will prolong life and it is not too burdensome, the duty is to use it even if the disease is incurable and the case is hopeless in that sense. One cannot simply argue that the disease is incurable and thus no obligation exists to preserve life, even if the patient is in what is called a persistent vegetative state.

Quality-of-Life Decisions

We are dealing with so-called quality-of-life decisions here. The principle underlying these decisions is that the duty to preserve life is based on quality of life. If one's life does not and will not meet a certain standard, it is not considered worth living or preserving. This would not justify taking positive measures to end one's life. But short of doing this, a patient does not have to worry about whether the means he or she forgoes are burdensome or useless to preserve life. Even if they are not burdensome and they will prolong life, the patient is not obliged to use them. The patient's duty to life is based on the quality of that life rather than on the nature of the means needed to preserve it. This article cannot treat this issue deeply. Suffice it to say here that appeal to quality of life as the reason for nontreatment goes beyond the traditional option regarding means and allows one to forgo even unburdensome and useful means of preserving life. In the traditional discernment of the duty to respect life, no distinction is made between taking positive measures to end life (suicide and homicide) and forgoing means that are not burdensome but useful to prolong life. Omission of such means (e.g., a hunger strike or starving a person) is not distinguished from taking positive measures to cause death. Both are condemned, and no allowance is made for quality-of-life considerations.

The defense brought in an expert in medical ethics, Rev. John J. Paris, SJ, as witness to the ethics of non-treatment in this case. Fr. Paris took the position that withdrawing the treatment in question was morally permissible in this case. He enumerated three cases in which this kind of nontreatment might be judged permissible:

1. The patient is brain dead.
2. The patient is terminally ill.
3. The patient is in a permanent coma.

I do not think anyone would dispute the first case. If the patient is brain dead, treatment becomes useless and hence cannot be obligatory. This is true even if one does not identify brain death with what might be called traditional death (cessation of heart and lung activity). Death is clearly imminent in these cases and will defy treatment. In other words, treatment will be useless; so nontreatment is morally permissible.

I think there would be agreement as well on the second case, depending on the meaning one gives to the term "terminally ill." If death is imminent whether the patient uses the treatment or not, the treatment again becomes useless. But Fr. Paris said in another part of his testimony that a terminal case was one in which the patient would die within a year. I am not sure that there would be agreement with his judgment on the second case, if "terminal" is understood in that sense. Generally speaking, "imminent" in this context means a short time (e.g., two weeks). If death is imminent in this sense, with or without treatment, the treatment would be considered useless and therefore not obligatory.

It is with the third case that I have serious difficulty. I think the fact that the patient is in a permanent coma would justify withdrawing excessively burdensome treatment, but I do not think it would justify withdrawing treatment that would be ordinary (unburdensome) but useful to prolong life. One who takes the position that it is permissible to withdraw all treatment when a person is in a permanent coma (or in a persistent vegetative state or with irreversible brain damage) is making quality of life the norm for the obligation to preserve life, and this goes beyond what has been traditionally allowed.

Fr. Paris takes the position that the quality of life of people in an irreversible coma, a persistent vegetative state, or with irreversible brain damage (he uses all three terms) is so low that there is no obligation to preserve it. Such an obligation would arise only if there were hope of restoring the person to consciousness. He objects to the charge that he is saying that life has no value in the above circumstances. What he is saying is that such patients (like Mr. Herbert) have exhausted their potential for value and for living. It would follow that since there is no potential for life, there is no obligation to it. I understand how one can say that a person who is dead has no potential for life, but I do not understand how one can say that a person who is actually living has no potential for life. If he is in an irreversible coma, he may have no potential for conscious life, but this is something else—unless one identifies life with conscious life. Unfortunately, Fr. Paris seems to be saying that, as far as the duty to preserve life goes, one has no more obligation to preserve (irreversibly) unconscious life than he has to death.

Prolonging Life Is a Benefit

Another observation about Fr. Paris's testimony may be pertinent. He gives the impression that the Vatican Congregation for the Doctrine of Faith's *Declaration on Euthanasia* (USCC, Washington, DC, 1980) abandoned the ordinary/extraordinary means distinction in favor of a distinction between proportionate and disproportionate means. A closer reading of this document will show that it merely points out that the former distinction causes confusion today and that some have substituted the latter distinction. The *Declaration* itself is more concerned about basic principles than verbal distinctions, and states clearly that the principles remain the same. As I have already pointed out, these principles refer to burden and benefit, or use. If a treatment is not burdensome and would be beneficial, it is considered a duty to use it. And prolonging life is considered a benefit. In fact, this is the assumption underlying the whole discussion. In no way does the *Declaration* make allowance for a sliding rule that would remove any obligation to preserve life in so-called hopeless cases. So it cannot be appealed to in support of this position.

Unfortunately, the judge of the Superior Court of Appeals in the Herbert case seemed to base his judgment on just such a rule. As he says, "A treatment course which is only minimally painful or intrusive may nonetheless be considered disproportionate to the potential benefits if the prognosis is virtually hopeless for any significant improvement in condition." The judge cites *Deciding to Forego Life-Sustaining Treatment* (President's Commission for the Study of Ethical Problems in Medicine and Biomedical and Behavioral Research, U.S. Government Printing Office, Washington, DC, 1983, pp. 82–90) as the source of this judgment.

One could accept this judgment for a terminally ill patient when treatment would be truly useless. Fr. Paris's testimony indeed contained much discussion of the question whether the patient was terminally ill, but this discussion did not turn out to be relevant to the final decision. As we have seen, Fr. Paris himself allowed withdrawal of treatment even for a nonterminally ill patient in an irreversible coma. And the judge based his decision on this norm. Since treatment would not return the patient to a sapient or cognitive state, it could be omitted even if the condition were not terminal. The fact that treatment would prolong life was not considered relevant. In other words, the judgment was based on quality of life. Whatever the judgment of the morality of treatment withdrawal in the Herbert case, I find it disturbing that the court decision is based on a quality-of-life judgment.

21

Caring or Starving? The Case of Claire Conroy

Richard A. McCormick, SJ

Claire Conroy was an eighty-four-year-old nursing home resident. She suffered from irreversible physical and mental impairments including arteriosclerotic heart disease, diabetes, and hypertension. She could neither speak nor swallow and was fed by a nasogastric tube. Her movements were very limited though she could smile or moan in response to some stimuli. She was restricted to a semi-fetal position and lacked control of her excretory functions. Thomas C. Whittemore, Miss Conroy's nephew and guardian, requested that the nasogastric tube be removed from his awake but severely demented aunt. The application was opposed by Miss Conroy's guardian "ad litem" (for purposes of litigation).

At trial, two physicians testified that Miss Conroy would die of dehydration in about a week after removal of the nasogastric tube. They also concurred in the opinion that her death would be painful. One physician regarded the nasogastric feeding as optional medical treatment. Miss Conroy's own physician, however, believed that removal of the tube would be unacceptable medical practice. The trial court (Judge Reginald Stanton, Feb. 2, 1983) decided to permit removal of the tube because Miss Conroy's life had become intolerably and permanently burdensome.

This decision was appealed by Miss Conroy's guardian ad litem, but she died while the appeal was pending. However, the appellate division considered the matter too important to be left unresolved. It reversed the trial court's judgment and stated that removal of the nasogastric tube would be tantamount to killing her. A guardian's decision, the court argued, may never be used to withhold nourishment from an incompetent patient. As the court worded it: "The trial judge authorized euthanasia [homicide]. . . . If the trial judge's order had been enforced, Conroy would not have died as the result of an existing medical condition, but rather she would have died, and painfully so, as the result of a new and independent condition: dehydration and starvation. Thus she would have been actively killed by independent means."

Mr. Whittemore took the question to the New Jersey Supreme Court, the same court that had decided the Karen Quinlan case. The court released its decision Jan. 17, 1985. After acknowledging the right of a competent adult to decline medical treatment—a right embraced within the common-law right of self-determination—the court addressed the rights of the incompetent. It noted: "The right of an adult who, like Claire Conroy, was once competent, to determine the course of her medical treatment remains intact even when she is no longer able to assert that right or to appreciate its effectuation."

Clearly a substitute decision-maker or proxy must be called upon to function at this point. May a proxy ever decide that life-sustaining treatment may be withheld or withdrawn from an incompetent but not comatose patient? The court responded in the affirmative and proposed three tests or standards corresponding to three different situations. First, there is the "subjective standard," under which life-sustaining treatment may be withheld or withdrawn "when it is *clear* that the particular patient would have refused the treatment under the circumstances involved" (emphasis added). This clear intent can be concluded from written directives (living will) or oral statements made to family, friends or health providers. It might also derive from a durable power of attorney or appointment of a proxy with authorization to make medical decisions on the patient's behalf.

Second, there is the "limited objective test." Life-sustaining treatment may be withheld or withdrawn from a patient like Claire Conroy when there is trustworthy evidence that the patient would have refused the treatment and the proxy is satisfied that the burdens of the patient's continued life with the treatment outweigh the benefits of that life for the patient.

Finally there is the "pure objective test." Under this test the burdens of the patient's life with treatment should clearly and markedly outweigh the benefits the patient derives from life. Furthermore, the unavoidable and severe pain of the patient's life with treatment must be such that continued life-sustaining treatment would be inhumane.

In elaborating its decision, which was a reversal of the appellate division's judgment that cessation of artificial feeding was a killing act, the New Jersey Supreme Court made several interesting points. First, it stated that the record in the Conroy case did not satisfy the standards prescribed by the opinion. Second, it rejected several distinctions as analytically unhelpful in this case: the distinction between actively hastening death and passively allowing a person to die; the distinction between withholding and withdrawing; the distinction between ordinary and extraordinary means. For instance, the court viewed the active–passive distinction as "elusive" and "particularly nebulous" where withholding or withdrawing life-sustaining treatment is concerned. It stated: "In a case like that of Claire Conroy, for example, would a physician who discontinued nasogastric feeding be actively causing her death by removing her primary source of nutrients; or would he merely be omitting to continue the artificial form of treatment, thus passively allowing her medical condition, which includes her inability to swallow, to take its natural course?"

Third, the court stated clearly that artificial feeding by nasogastric tube or intravenous infusion is equivalent to artificial breathing by a respirator. In other words, it is a medical procedure and should be provided or withheld according to the criteria applicable to medical procedures.

Finally and very importantly, it stipulated a procedure to be followed in cases like that of Claire Conroy. The person (e.g., family member, guardian, physician) who believes that withholding or withdrawing life-sustaining treatment corresponds to the patient's wishes or would be in her/his best interests must notify an ombudsman. Those with contrary beliefs should do the same. The ombudsman is to treat every such notification of withholding or withdrawing as a possible abuse. Two physicians unaffiliated with the nursing home and with the attending physician must confirm the patient's medical condition and prognosis.

This decision is, in a sense, a linear descendent of a previous case involving withdrawing or feeding. Clarence Herbert underwent surgery for closure of an ileostomy at Kaiser Permanente Hospital, Harbor City, Calif., in 1981. Shortly after successful completion of the surgery, Herb suffered cardiorespiratory arrest. He was revived and immediately placed on life-support equipment. Within the following three days it was determined that Mr. Herbert was in a deeply comatose state from which he was unlikely to recover. Tests performed by several physicians indicated that he had suffered severe brain damage, leaving him in a vegetative state that was likely to be permanent.

At that time Mr. Herbert's physicians, Dr. Robert Nejdl and Dr. Neil Barber, informed his family of his condition and the extremely poor prognosis. The family then drafted a written request to the hospital personnel stating that they wanted "all machines taken off that are sustaining life." Dr. Nejdl and Dr. Barber complied and removed Mr. Herbert from the respirator. He continued to breathe. After two more days, the two physicians, after consulting with the family (though the record is a bit hazy here), ordered removal of the intravenous line and nasogastric tube that provided hydration and nourishment. Shortly thereafter Mr. Herbert died.

Dr. Nejdl and Dr. Barber were accused of murder by the Los Angeles District Attorney. Los Angeles Municipal Judge Brian Crahan dismissed the case. It was reopened (May 5, 1983) by Superior Court Judge Robert A. Wenke on the grounds that the dismissal was erroneous. The Herbert case received widespread publicity. The implications of Judge Wenke's decision were stated simply by Dr. Barber: "No doctor will take a patient off a respirator now."

The matter eventually reached the Court of Appeal. On Oct. 12, 1983, Judge Lynn Compton exonerated Dr. Nejdl and Dr. Barber of any unlawful conduct. In the course of this opinion, the court made several interesting and important points. First, Judge Compton noted that even though life-support devices are self-propelled, still each drop of IV fluid is "comparable to a manually administered injection or item of medication." Hence disconnecting such devices is "comparable to withholding the manually administered injection." Second, the court viewed intravenous nourishment and fluid as "being the same as the use of the respirator." Third, medical nutrition and hydration resemble medical procedures rather than typical ways of providing nutrition and hydration. Hence they are to be evaluated in terms of their burdens and benefits. Finally, since the court viewed the physicians' actions as omissions rather than affirmative actions, the resolution of the case depends on whether there was a duty to continue to provide life-sustaining treatment. The court asserted that there is no such duty once the treatment is useless. And it was useless in Herbert's case because it merely sustained biological life with no realistic hope of a return to a cognitive, sapient state. Thus, continued use of life sustainers was "disproportionate."

These two cases have a key difference. Clarence Herbert was judged to be in a permanent vegetative state. Claire Conroy was not. She was incompetent but not comatose. Of those in a permanent vegetative state, the President's Commission for the Study of Ethical Problems in Medicine and Biomedical and

Behavioral Research wrote in *Decisions to Forgo Life-Sustaining Treatment*, 1983, 190: "Most patients with permanent unconsciousness cannot be sustained for long without an array of increasingly artificial feeding interventions—nasogastric tubes, gastrostomy tubes, or intravenous nutrition. Since permanently unconscious patients will never be aware of nutrition, the only benefit to the patient of providing such increasingly burdensome interventions is sustaining the body to allow for a remote possibility of recovery. The sensitivities of the family and of care-giving professionals ought to determine whether such interventions are made."

A footnote to this last sentence notes that it can be anticipated that courts will grant requests to withhold or withdraw further treatment, including IV drips, from such patients. And that is just what the court did in the Herbert case. But the New Jersey Supreme Court also did the same thing in principle in the Conroy case, and for some of the same reasons. That is, both courts regard feeding by IV lines and nasogastric tubes as basically medical procedures to be judged by a burdens–benefits calculus. Furthermore, both courts (to a lesser degree the New Jersey Supreme Court) allow "quality-of-life" components to function in determining the best interests of the patient.

There is another feature of these decisions that could easily be missed. Both represent reversals of lower courts that held that withholding or withdrawing nutrition-hydration from comatose and/or incompetent patients would constitute murder. I think it fair to say that these judicial disagreements reflect the state of ethical discussion that preceded them and still surrounds them.

One of the first shots in this discussion was fired by hospice nurse Joyce V. Zerwekh. She argued in *Nursing*, January 1983, that it is not always more merciful to administer IV fluids to a dying patient. There are both beneficial and detrimental effects associated with dehydration and the judgment must be individualized.

Since the Zerwekh study, the literature has piled up impressively. For instance, Kenneth Micetich, MD, Patricia Steinecker, MD, and ethicist David Thomasma (all of Stritch School of Medicine, Loyola University, Chicago) concurred that IV fluids may not be morally required under a threefold condition: (1) The patient must be dying. "Death will be imminent (within two weeks) no matter what intervention we may take"; (2) The patient must be comatose. Comatose patients would experience no pain, thirst, etc.; and (3) The family must request that no further medical procedures be done in the face of impending death (*Archives of Internal Medicine*, 1983).

James Childress, of the University of Virginia, and Joanne Lynn, MD, of George Washington University, carried the matter a step further. They argued that there are cases, even though relatively few, when it is in the best interests of patients to be malnourished and dehydrated. They listed three situations: (1) The procedures that would be required could be considered futile; (2) The improvement in nutritional and fluid balance, though achievable, could be of no benefit to the patient (e.g., persistent vegetative state); and (3) There are cases where the burdens to be borne in receiving the treatment may outweigh the benefit. Terminal pulmonary edema, nausea and mental confusion may be more likely in some patients as a result of artificial hydration and nutrition (*Hastings Center Report*, October 1983).

Even more recently a group of distinguished clinicians advocated the withholding of parenteral fluids and nutritional support from severely and irrevocably demented patients and, occasionally, from elderly patients with permanent mild impairment of competence, a group characterized as "pleasantly senile" (*New England Journal of Medicine*, 1984).

Such voices have not gone unchallenged. Daniel Callahan (*Hastings Center*) agrees that it is morally licit to discontinue feeding in the circumstances noted by Lynn and Childress. Yet he is profoundly uneasy with that conclusion. The feeding of the hungry, whether they be poor or physically unable to feed themselves, is "the most fundamental of all human relationships" (*Hastings Center Report*, October 1983). It is, he argues, extremely dangerous to tamper with so central a moral emotion. There remains a deep-seated revulsion at stopping feeding even under legitimate circumstances. As I read him, Mr. Callahan would respect that revulsion and continue feeding as "a tolerable price to pay to preserve—with ample margin to spare—one of the few moral emotions that could just as easily be called a necessary social instinct."

Gilbert Meilaender of Oberlin College carries this a step further. He argues that the withdrawal of nourishment from permanently unconscious patients involves us in "aiming at their deaths." This we should never do. Nor does their permanent comatose state mean that it is useless to feed them. In these cases, feeding remains care for the embodied person, and it is dualistic to think otherwise. Nor is the care "in any strict sense medical treatment." It treats no particular disease; rather "it gives what all need to live" (*Hastings Center Report*, December 1984).

A physician (Mark Siegler) and an attorney (Alan J. Weisbard) are deeply troubled by the emerging literature justifying withholding or withdrawing of hydration and nutritional support (*Archives of Internal Medicine*, January 1985). They reject the idea that anyone (physicians, families, courts) can properly make such judgments for the incompetent. Therefore, they want to reverse the stream of this literature and offer several arguments to bolster this reversal. First, patients will be protected against diagnostic errors, inadequate treatment and unscrupulous (e.g., for financial reasons) care. Second, physicians will not be compelled to make ad hoc, quality-of-life judgments. Third, the medical profession will be protected against the gradual dilution of its dedication to the welfare of patients. Finally, society will benefit by rejecting this practice because it bears the seeds of unacceptable consequences (e.g., devaluation of the unproductive).

This is a sampling of the literature that preceded and still surrounds the Claire Conroy decision. Where does it leave us? With several key issues and a final caution.

1. *The notion of a dying patient.* Who would be said to be a dying patient? If a patient needs dialysis to survive, is that patient a dying or nondying patient? If one needs a respirator to survive and will die without it, is that person dying or not? If one needs a nasogastric tube or a gastrostomy for food intake, is that person dying or not? I am suggesting that the notion of "the dying patient" is ambiguous and sometimes related to the technology available. However, the category is often presented as if it were utterly clear. This is a key issue; for if a patient is said to be nondying, but dies as a result of nutrient-withdrawal, then that withdrawal appears to be positively causal, and the withdrawer a killer.

2. *The nature of artificial hydration-nutrition.* Is this most properly characterized as a medical procedure, as both the appeals court of California and the New Jersey Supreme Court, as well as much of the literature, contend? Or does it more closely resemble providing a person with a bowl of soup? Does the simple fact that artificial feeding "gives what all need to live" (Meilaender) imply that how it is given makes no difference in its description? Most of us would not know how to go about providing nutrition and hydration by nasogastric tube and IV lines. These procedures require skilled medical training. Does that not constitute them strictly medical procedures? This is an issue because normal feeding has profound symbolic importance in human relationships and societal structure. It is one thing to starve the hungry. We should be appalled at the idea. It is quite another to withhold or withdraw a medical procedure. That we do routinely, and justifiably.

Whether artificial nutrition and hydration are medical procedures or not is often confused by the introduction of terms such as hunger and thirst. People can be denied artificial nutrition and hydration without experiencing hunger and thirst. Conversely, they can feel hunger and thirst without being malnourished or dehydrated. The usage "feed the hungry and thirsty" in this context tends to predispose us to regard artificial nutrition and hydration as something other than medical procedures.

3. *The intention of death.* When we withdraw nutrition and hydration from a permanently comatose patient, must we be said to be "aiming at death" (Meilaender)? The answer to this question will depend very closely on how we answer the first two. For example, if permanently comatose patients or profoundly incompetent ones are said to be dying patients (because their condition prevents normal ingestion of food, e.g., swallowing) and if artificial feeding by nasogastric tube is to be regarded as a medical procedure, then withdrawal of nutrients represents only omission of a medical procedure for a dying patient. This need not involve "aiming at death"; otherwise any such omission (e.g., of a respirator) would in principle involve this reprehensible intent.

On the other hand, if the patient is viewed as nondying, and artificial provision of nutrients is not a medical procedure but rather an instance of "normal, ordinary care," then omission of such nutrients could be more suspect.

Let me put it this way. Those who contend that withdrawing hydration and nutrition involves us in "aiming death" or being involved in "the direct causal responsibility for death" (Siegler, Weisbard) must be consistent and apply their analysis to the competent patient. Is a competent patient who refuses a nasogastric tube or a gastrostomy guilty of suicide ("aiming at his own death")? Most of us would and should answer: "It all depends." If the patient can be tided over a transitory illness and returned to normal life, the treatment would surely be obligatory and refusal of it, other things being equal, would be suicidal. If, however, this is not the case and the artificial feeding is foreseeably permanent, the treatment would be morally optional. Being such, it would not necessarily involve a death-aim. It need involve only a thoroughly Christian assertion that there are values greater in life than living, that we all retain the right to decide how we shall live while dying.

4. *The burden–benefit calculus.* Where medical procedures are in question, it is generally admitted that the criterion to be used is a burdens–benefits estimate. This was the criterion proposed by the Sacred Congregation for the Doctrine of Faith in its *Declaration on Euthanasia* (May 5, 1980) and by the President's commission. The question posed is: Will the burden of the treatment outweigh the

benefits to the patient? The general answer: If the treatment is useless or futile, or if it imposes burdens that outweigh the benefits, it may be omitted.

However, an ambiguity remains. What is to count as a burden, and correlatively as a benefit? If a patient's life can be prolonged, but only in a comatose state, is that a benefit to the patient? Or if treatment will preserve life, but only a pain-racked, incompetent life, is that a benefit?

The issue here is this: In weighing the burdens–benefits of a treatment, is it the burden of the treatment only (e.g., its pain, expense etc.) that is legitimately considered, or may we include in the assessment the burden of continued existence itself? In other words, may the quality of life preserved be a proper dimension of the calculus?

The President's commission answered this last question in the affirmative when it defined the patient's best interest broadly to "take into account such factors as the relief of suffering, the preservation or restoration of functioning, and the quality as well as the extent of the life sustained." Both the Herbert court and the Conroy court did the same. For instance, the Conroy court (New Jersey Supreme Court) acknowledged that "although we are condoning a restricted evaluation of the nature of a patient's life in terms of pain, suffering, and possible enjoyment under the limited-objective and pure objective tests, we expressly decline to authorize decision-making based on assessments of the personal worth or social utility of another's life, or the value of that life to others."

Some continue to attempt to finesse this extremely difficult and delicate issue by conceptualizing decisions in terms of "ordinary" and "extraordinary" means. But it will not work. Such terms only disguise the quality-of-life component unavoidably present in some of these decisions. For this reason nearly every recent commentator would agree with the President's commission when it stated: "The claim, then that the treatment is extraordinary is more of an expression of the conclusion than a justification for it."

My own opinion on these issues is that the permanently comatose and *some* noncomatose but elderly incompetent patients may be classified broadly as dying; that feeding by IV lines and nasogastric tubes is a medical procedure; that its discontinuance need not involve aiming at the death of such patients; and that the burden–benefit calculus may include, indeed often unavoidably includes, a quality-of-life ingredient, providing we draw the line at the right place.

And that brings us to the caution. The Claire Conroy case and the decision of the New Jersey Supreme Court may appear to be isolated instances. That is not the case. There are many thousands of nursing home residents like Claire Conroy. They are a terribly vulnerable population. They are elderly and often suffer from crippling disabilities. They often are without surviving relatives. Physicians play a more limited role in nursing homes than in hospitals, and patient advocacy is correspondingly less intense. Furthermore, as the New Jersey Supreme Court notes, nursing homes are often afflicted with industry-wide problems that make them a very troubled and troublesome component of the health care system. And all of this at the very time when there are economic and social pressures on health care delivery. Together these factors may make it extremely difficult to keep patients' best interests at the heart of these decisions. In other words, the potential for abuse is enormous.

This suggests the wisdom of Daniel Callahan's statement at a spring conference on these problems in 1984: "The time to curtail abuses in the future is to begin now in trying to go through those steps that will draw lines very carefully." We have moved from Quinlan (persistent vegetative state—removal of respirator) to Herbert (persistent vegetative state—removal of respirator, nasogastric tube, and IV lines) to Conroy (incompetent but noncomatose—removal of nasogastric tube). The progression is obvious, and obviously dangerous, unless we draw clear lines based on clear criteria. If we do not, we will not long be confined within the limits set forth in cases like Conroy.

Technology can help us or hurt us, individually and societally, and in ways that are awesome in their implications. The recent technological revolution in methods of hydration and nutritional maintenance is a case in point. That is why the ultimate caution was well stated by the New Jersey Supreme Court: When evidence of a person's wishes is equivocal, or the best interests determination doubtful, "it is best to err, if at all, in favor of preserving life."

Permissions

We gratefully acknowledge permission to reprint the following material.

Chapter 1. American Academy of Neurology, "Position of the American Academy of Neurology on Certain Aspects of the Care and Management of the Persistent Vegetative State Patient," *Neurology* 39 (January, 1989): 125–26.

Chapter 2. Myles N. Sheehan, SJ, "Feeding Tubes: Sorting Out the Issues," *Health Progress* 82 (November–December, 2001): 22–27. © 2001 by the Catholic Health Association. Reproduced from *Health Progress* with permission.

Chapter 3. Michael R. Panicola, "Catholic Teaching on Prolonging Life: Setting the Record Straight," *Hastings Center Report* 31 (November–December, 2001): 14–25.

Chapter 4. Donald E. Henke, "A History of Ordinary and Extraordinary Means," Reprinted from *The National Catholic Bioethics Quarterly* 5.3 (Autumn 2005): 555–75. © 2005 The National Catholic Bioethics Center. All rights reserved. Used with permission.

Chapter 5. Ronald Hamel and Michael Panicola, "Must We Preserve Life?" *America* 190 (April 19–26, 2004): 6–13. For subscription information, call 1-800-627-9533 or visit www.americamagazine.org.

Chapter 6. Pope Pius XII, "The Prolongation of Life," *The Pope Speaks* 4 (Spring 1958): 393–98. Reprinted with permission of Liberia Editrice Vaticana.

Chapter 7. Sacred Congregation for the Doctrine of the Faith, "Declaration on Euthanasia," *Origins* 10 (August 14, 1980): 154–56. Reprinted with the permission of Libreria Editrice Vaticana.

Chapter 8. Pontifical Academy of Sciences, "The Artificial Prolongation of Life," *Origins* 15 (December 5, 1985): 415. Reprinted with permission of Liberia Editrice Vaticana.

Chapter 9. Texas Bishops and The Texas Conference of Catholic Health Facilities, "On Withdrawing Artificial Nutrition and Hydration," *Origins* 20 (June 7, 1990): 53–55. Reprinted with permission of the Texas Catholic Conference.

Chapter 10. National Conference of Catholic Bishops' Committee for Pro-Life Activities, "Nutrition and Hydration: Moral and Pastoral Reflections," Washington, DC: National Conference of Catholic Bishops, 1992.

Chapter 11. United States Conference of Catholic Bishops, "Ethical and Religious Directives, Introduction to Part V and Directives 57–58," Washington, DC: United States Conference of Catholic Bishops, 2001.

Chapter 12. Thomas A. Shannon and James J. Walter, "The PVS Patient and the Forgoing/Withdrawing of Medical Nutrition and Hydration," *Theological Studies* 49 (December, 1988): 623–47.

Chapter 13. Germain Grisez, "Should Nutrition and Hydration Be Provided to Permanently Unconscious and Other Mentally Disabled Persons?" *Linacre Quarterly* 57 (May, 1990): 30–43.

Chapter 14. Daniel P. Sulmasy, OFM, "End of Life Care Revisited," *Health Progress* 87 (July–August, 2006): 50–56. © 2006 by the Catholic Health Association. Reproduced from *Health Progress* with permission.

Chapter 15. Pope John Paul II, "Care for Patients in a 'Permanent' Vegetative State," *Origins* 33 (April 8, 2004): 737, 739–40. Reprinted with the permission of Libreria Editrice Vaticana.

Chapter 16. Richard Doerflinger, "John Paul II on the 'Vegetative State'." Reprinted from *Ethics & Medics* 29.6 (June 2004): 2–4. © 2004. The National Catholic Bioethics Center. All rights reserved. Used with permission.

Chapter 17. Mark Repenshek and John Paul Slosar, "Medically Assisted Nutrition and Hydration: A Contribution to the Dialogue," *Hastings Center Report* 34 (November–December, 2004): 13–16.

Chapter 18. Thomas A. Shannon and James J. Walter, "Assisted Nutrition and Hydration and the Catholic Tradition," *Theological Studies* 66 (September, 2005): 651–62.

Chapter 19. Kevin O'Rourke, OP, "Reflections on the Papal Allocution Concerning Care for Persistent Vegetative State Patients," *Christian Bioethics* 12 (April, 2006): 83–97. © 2006 From *Christian Bioethics* by Kevin O'Rourke. Reproduced by permission of Taylor & Francis Group, LLC., http://www.taylorandfrancis.com.

Chapter 20. John R. Connery, SJ, "The Clarence Herbert Case: Was Withdrawal of Treatment Justified?" *Hospital Progress* 65 (February, 1984): 32–35, 70. © 1984 by the Catholic Health Association. Reproduced from *Hospital Progress* with permission.

Chapter 21. Richard A. McCormick, SJ, "Caring or Starving? The Case of Claire Conroy," *America* 152 (April 6, 1985): 269–73. For subscription information, call 1-800-627-9533 or visit www.americamagazine.org.

Contributors

American Academy of Neurology

John R. Connery, SJ, was professor of theology at Loyola University Chicago.

Richard Doerflinger is adjunct fellow, National Catholic Bioethics Center and deputy director, Secretariat for Pro-Life Activities at the U.S. Conference of Catholic Bishops.

Germain Grisez is professor of moral theology at Mount Saint Mary College, Emmitsburg, Maryland.

Ronald Hamel is senior director for ethics of the Catholic Health Association, St. Louis, Missouri.

Donald E. Henke is associate dean and assistant professor of moral theology at Kenrick-Glennon Seminary in St. Louis, Missouri.

Pope John Paul II was pontiff from 1978 to 2005.

Richard A. McCormick, SJ, was professor of moral theology, University of Notre Dame, Indiana.

National Conference of Catholic Bishops' Committee for Pro-Life Activities

Kevin O'Rourke, OP, is a professor in the Neiswanger Institute of Bioethics and Health Policy, Stritch School of Medicine, Loyola University Chicago.

Michael R. Panicola is vice president of ethics for SSM Health Care, St. Louis, Missouri.

Pope Pius XII was pontiff from 1939 to 1958.

Pontifical Academy of Sciences

Mark Repenshek is health care ethicist, Columbia St. Mary's, Milwaukee, Wisconsin.

Sacred Congregation for the Doctrine of the Faith

Thomas A. Shannon taught ethics at Worcester Polytechnic Institute in Worcester, Massachusetts, before his retirement.

Myles N. Sheehan, SJ, is senior associate dean, Education Program Administration and associate professor of medicine/geriatrics at Loyola University Chicago.

John Paul Slosar is the director of ethics for Ascension Health in St. Louis, Missouri.

Daniel P. Sulmasy, OFM, holds the John J. Conley Chair in Ethics at St. Vincent's Hospital, Manhattan, and is professor of medical ethics at the New York Medical College, Valhalla, New York.

Texas Bishops and the Texas Conference of Catholic Health Facilities

United States Conference of Catholic Bishops

James J. Walter is the Austin & Ann O'Malley Professor of Bioethics and chair of The Bioethics Institute at Loyola Marymount University in Los Angeles.

Index